Would You Like To Know . . .

- What foods to eat for optimum health?
- High or low protein diet – which is better?
- How arthritis and cancer are cured in Europe?
- The truth about the nutrition-sex relationship?
- What is the real cause of baldness?
- How to fast – and how not to?
- Is milk a friend or a fiend?
- Should you take vitamins and food supplements?
- Must you drink distilled water?
- How to protect yourself against polluted air?
- Should you eat meat?
- What can fermented foods do for your health?
- How can certain health foods harm you?
- The truth about rejuvenating herbs?
- Why is vitamin X called "Youth Vitamin"?
- How do overheating therapies cure "incurable" diseases?
- Can aging be prevented or postponed?
- What is health and rejuvenation secret number one?

Are you CONFUSED on these and other pertinent questions related to nutrition, health and longevity?

In the following chapters you will find *factual answers to these and many, many other controversial questions.* The answers may surprise, startle – even shock you. If only one of the answers, suggestions and tips offered in this book can help to De-CONFUSE your mind and lead you to better health and longer life, then you will be richly rewarded for the effort of reading it.

Dedicated to all earnest and sincere seekers of better health

ACKNOWLEDGEMENT

I wish to express my deep and lasting appreciation to Dr. Leslie H. Salov, M.D., and to my many friends and assistants who have helped in the preparation of this book.

Paavo O. Airola

Are You Confused?

DE-CONFUSION BOOK ON NUTRITION & HEALTH,
with the latest scientific research and
authoritative answers to the most
controversial questions

by PAAVO O. AIROLA, N.D., Ph.D.

FOREWORD by LESLIE H. SALOV, M.D.

HEALTH PLUS, PUBLISHERS
P. O. BOX 22001, PHOENIX, ARIZONA 85028

ARE YOU CONFUSED?

ISBN 0-932090-04-4
HARD COVER PRINTING, JANUARY, 1971
SECOND LARGE PRINTING,
PAPERBACK EDITION, AUGUST, 1972
THIRD PRINTING, OCTOBER, 1974
FOURTH PRINTING, OCTOBER, 1975
FIFTH PRINTING, MAY, 1976
SIXTH PRINTING, OCTOBER, 1976
SEVENTH PRINTING, MARCH, 1977
EIGHTH PRINTING, SEPTEMBER, 1977
NINTH PRINTING, JUNE, 1978
TENTH PRINTING, FEBRUARY, 1979
ELEVENTH PRINTING, DECEMBER, 1979
TWELFTH PRINTING, OCTOBER, 1980

By the same author:

HOW TO GET WELL
REJUVENATION SECRETS FROM AROUND THE WORLD — THAT "WORK"
HOW TO KEEP SLIM, HEALTHY AND YOUNG WITH JUICE FASTING
CANCER: CAUSES, PREVENTION AND TREATMENT — THE TOTAL APPROACH
SWEDISH BEAUTY SECRETS
STOP HAIR LOSS
THERE IS A CURE FOR ARTHRITIS
HEALTH SECRETS FROM EUROPE
SEX AND NUTRITION
THE MIRACLE OF GARLIC
EVERYWOMAN'S BOOK

printed in the U.S.A.

Foreword

by Leslie H. Salov, M.D.

People are seeking pathways to good health in many ways: they put themselves under the care of medical doctors, osteopaths, naturopaths, chiropractors, psychologists, psychiatrists . . . Some who seek professional care and do not improve try to help themselves with various self-treatments and health programs. They buy health foods by the load, vitamins, wheat grass juices; they go on fat-free, sugar-free, or low-calorie diets; they exercise, they jog, they sprint, they walk, they do yoga . . . etc., etc.

Many people, after trying to get help from medical doctors and from the other healing professions and not getting any improvement, are dissatisfied and completely *confused* as to where to turn for the real answers to their health problems.

Confusion is present not only among those who are sick, but also among the various healing professions. Sometimes the methods of treatment in these professions are diametrically opposed, starting from different hypotheses and contradictory theories of the causes of disease.

The confused public has the right to demand the reliable information on the vital topics of health and the scientifically proven therapies to treat the growing number of sick people.

Dr. Paavo O. Airola, in this book, *ARE YOU CONFUSED?* does an excellent job of helping to *"de-confuse"* the confused reader about the many questions pertaining to health, and particularly pertaining to nutrition. The task he has taken upon himself is tremendous and his book is complete and extremely useful to everyone.

In Chapter 14, *Biological Medicine – the Healing Science of Tomorrow,* which particularly appeals to me, the author visualizes a new, glorious era when all the healing professions will be united in one complete and perfect healing system – *Biological Medicine.* New biological medical schools will teach future doctors all the known arts of healing: allopathic, naturopathic, chiropractic, herbal, homeopathic, psychosomatic, spiritual, etc. Biological Medicine will stress the preventive approach to disease. Its philosophy is based on the fundamental principle of intelligent co-operation with nature and of assisting the body's own inherent healing powers with all the available harmless and effective therapies – be they drugs, surgery, vitamins, controlled or improved nutrition, manipulations, herbs or a psychological or spiritual approach. Biological Medicine will also consider the important part the mind plays in sickness and health.

Biological Medicine will be particularly concerned with the importance of nutrition in health and disease; the great benefits of organic farming; the danger of poisons in air, water and foods; and the ways and means of preventing and correcting the problems of environmental pollution.

The new Healing Science will take care of the total man, his spirit, his mind, and his body. The Doctor of Biological Medicine will teach people the correct ways of living to prevent disease and attain optimum health.

Dr. Airola's book is an important milestone on the road to the realization of this new concept of the perfect science of preventing and healing disease – Biological Medicine. However, before this can become a reality, the "de-confusion" among the healing professions, as well as among the confused health-conscious laymen, on the multitude of controversial questions related to health, nutrition, and various healing methods, is imperative. This book offers invaluable help in this "de-confusion" process.

Leslie H. Salov, M.D.
Director,
Athena Center for Creative Living

Introduction

Widespread Confusion

Miss Bea B., on her second visit to my office, walked to my desk holding two of my books, *HEALTH SECRETS FROM EUROPE* and *THERE IS A CURE FOR ARTHRITIS,* and said enthusiastically:

"Doctor, before you do anything, I want to tell you something. I just finished reading your books and for the first time in my life I am beginning to see the light. For the last twenty or so years I have been reading health books and health magazines, and listening to health lectures. And the more I read and listened to all the so-called experts and authorities, the more confused I became. Every book, every magazine article, and every authority gives different advice, and points out a different road to better health. Sometimes in the same magazine issue there are two or more contradictory articles on the same topic. Just before I found your books, I was so disgusted with all the disagreement among the "experts" that I was thinking of giving up all my search for the real truth, and just eating what I like. Your books made real sense to me. How different from everything I have read before! You report facts, not just express your own beliefs and opinions."

And then, after catching her breath, she said:

"Why don't you write a new book and straighten out some of the confusion we all have on so many, many important topics? For instance, the protein confusion! So many writers advise lots of protein – the more, the better. Yet, after eating a high-protein diet all these years I – and most of my health-foodist friends – are only getting sicker and sicker. There are so many other questions we are completely confused about – like fasting. Is it harmful or not? And what are the right and wrong ways to fast? Also, which is better – distilled water or purified spring water? Are wheat and milk really harmful? Or, should we take vitamins and supplements, or can we get all we need from the foods we eat? And so on, and so on."

This plea by Miss Bea B. to disperse her total confusion on so many vital questions of health and nutrition triggered my decision to write this DE-CONFUSION Book.

Desperate need

For the last several years I have gradually become aware of the desperate need for such a book. On my recent lecture and seminar tour in California and Arizona, I was appalled to find that so very few of my listeners – although most of them were veteran health-seekers – were enjoying perfect health, vibrant vitality, and freedom from disease. These sincere seekers of truth, well-read and health-educated, filled with health information far above the average American level, were religiously applying the knowledge they had acquired to improve their health. Yet, the hoped-for results of this application were missing. To my direct question to show by raising their hands how many could claim one hundred per cent glowing health, only a couple of reluctant hands went up in a several-hundred-strong audience.

Millions of people in the United States alone are what is popularly known as "health faddists". They are dedicated to improving their health through better nutrition and better living habits. They read bookshelves full of books and attend lectures. They support the fast-growing billion-dollar health food industry by buying all the acclaimed "miracle wonder-foods". They spend a fortune on vitamins, minerals, special food supplements, organic foods and high-protein powders. *Why, then, can so few of them claim perfect health and freedom from disease?*

For many years and in many countries I have heard the following comment when I advised someone to go to a health food store or hear a health lecture:

"I went to health lectures once, and I have been to health food stores, but I can tell you I have never seen so many sick-looking and emaciated people in all my life!"

For years I had a standard answer to such critics:

"The reason you see so many sick people in health food stores is not that *health foods made them sick,* but that only sick people are interested in health and health foods. You see, people are not interested in health until it starts to elude them. After running the usual course – doctors, drugs and hospitals – and becoming sicker and sicker, finally those who see the light decide to take their health into their own hands, and, as a last resort, become patrons of health food stores. That's why the average health food store customer is not the best picture of health."

However, I am becoming more and more doubtful about the completeness and correctness of the above answer. It is true, of course, that most health food store customers are sick in one or more ways. But I am beginning to encounter more and more people who have been trying for years to restore their health with health foods and supplements and are still not very healthy. And often, even previously healthy individuals, after years of eating health foods, become sick or are laking energy and vitality. Why?

Ignorance and Confusion

When recently the U. S. Department of Agriculture study, which showed that almost half of the American people were malnourished, was revealed, startled newsmen asked:

"What is the reason for this appalling paradox? How, in the country with the most abundant food supply in the world, can half of the people be undernourished or malnourished?"

The Assistant Secretary of Agriculture replied:

"Because of ignorance! People just don't know which foods they should eat. They spend their dollars on nutritionless foods and deprive themselves of health-building foods."

Although this may shock many a sincere health-seeker, the above answer can be used also to reply to the question: Why are many of the honest and dedicated seekers of health through better diet and food supplements not achieving the glowing health they are so earnestly striving for? *Ignorance,* and I will add, *confusion.*

During my lectures and seminars I see thousands of earnest health-seekers who are quite ignorant, and utterly confused, as to the *right ways and means* to improve their health and prevent disease.

The reason for this confusion is THE DIFFICULTY IN OBTAINING ABSOLUTELY RELIABLE, OBJECTIVE AND SCIENTIFICALLY CORRECT INFORMATION ON THE MOST VITAL QUESTIONS RELATED TO HEALTH, AND PARTICULARLY RELATED TO NUTRITION.

You read dozens of health books, attend lecture after lecture, read health magazine articles, consult the nutrition "experts" and authorities – *and you become only more and more confused.* Every book, every lecturer and every authority gives you *different answers* and points out *different roads* to glorious health.

One will tell you that the vegetarian diet will solve all your health problems – the other, that you will starve on a vegetarian diet and that you should eat lots of protein, especially meat.

One will advise you to take vitamins and food supplements – the other, that all isolated vitamins and supplements are "bad for you", and that you should get all your nutrients from the natural foods.

One will tell you that the ultimate answer to your health problems is raw, natural, organic, unprocessed foods, free from poisonous sprays and additives – the other that there is nothing wrong with foods available at the regular American supermarket, and that the only poisons to fear are those in the pens of the alarmist health writers!

These are only a few samples of hundreds of claims and theories proclaimed by vociferous titled and untitled authorities. *No wonder you are confused!*

This book is a direct answer to many urgent requests by sincere health-seekers for correct and reliable information on vital topics of health and nutrition. As you will see from the following chapters, this book is not just another book among hundreds that will confuse you even more. What I am going to tell you will not be my own beliefs or beautiful theories based on wishful thinking. I would not leave such an important matter as health of other people to the whim of my personal beliefs, prejudices, or likes. I have learned early in my life how dangerous it can be to have a dogmatic attitude when dealing with man's health. Thousands of people have been hurt and suffered because some great men made great mistakes in their calculations and conclusions. They based their conclusions on theories and wishful thinking, rather than facts.

Sources of information you can trust.

How can you trust that the advice and information you receive in this book are true scientific facts, and not just theories and beliefs? I have two great and dependable scientific sources on which I rely to corroborate my own conclusions:

1. The International Society for Research on Nutrition and Diseases of Civilization. Founded by Dr. Albert Schweitzer, the Society is comprised of several hundreds of foremost researchers and scientists from 75 countries – medical doctors, nutritionists, bio-chemists, and doctors of natural sciences. *The Society is absolutely independent in its research and actions.* It is not attached to or supported by industry or by professional or economic interests, or by any government. The list of the Scientific Council of this society reads like Who's Who in Science. It includes a great number of Nobel Prize Winners: the famous Vitamin C discoverer, Dr. A. Szent-Gyorgyi; the great Finnish scientist, Dr. A. I. Virtanen; American professor and biochemist Linus Pauling; world-famous Czechoslovakian researcher, Dr. J. Bernašek; Swedish scientist, Dr. K. H. Karström; American doctors B. W. Billow, R. M. Atwater, Max Warmbrand, etc. The recommendations and conclusions made by the Society are the results of the independent research and united consensus of all these great men of science.

The Society conducts and compiles research on nutrition and other environmental factors as they relate to man's health. For example, after seven years of research and study, it has worked out a recommendation for a *Macrobiotic Diet,* a diet most conductive to health and long life.

Don't you think that in today's labyrinth of conflicting ideas and opinions in the field of nutrition, the united opinion of this large and totally objective and independent scientific forum is more to be trusted than the subjective opinions of self-appointed health lecturers, writers and nutritionists, or the conclusions of the scattered research groups financed by the chemical and food-processing industries?

2. My second source of information is the EMPIRICAL evidence of centuries and milleniums of actual application.

Laboratory research and animal tests are only of limited value as compared to the thousands of years of actual human experience with nutrition capable of producing superior health.

Such empirical evidence is readily available. Dr. Sir Robert McCarrison, Dr. Weston Price, Arnold DeVries and other investigators, have traveled extensively, studying the living and the eating habits of peoples and tribes around the world known for their excellent health and freedom from disease. They have all concluded that the eating habits of these peoples are largely responsible for their superior health.

Based on these two superior sources of reliable information and corroborated by my own experience and the available data from recent research in various research centers of Germany, Russia and Sweden, this book will attempt to straighten out some of the most common misconceptions, myths, fallacies and half-truths concerning the vital questions related to nutrition and health.

One last note. Because of space limitations and the desire to make this a short and easily-read book, the presentation in this work is free from the usual references. I could have easily filled 25 pages or more with various references to substantiate every claim made. Those readers who are impressed by such voluminous references I advise to read my other works, which are richly documented, such as *HEALTH SECRETS FROM EUROPE, THERE IS A CURE FOR ARTHRITIS* and *NUTRITION AND SEX.* They contain the documented sources of scientific references for most of the claims presented in this book.

Table of Contents

Chapter 1

Why Universal Disagreement?

As I pointed out in the Introduction, there is total disagreement among various experts and authorities on many pertinent questions related to nutrition and health. You may wonder, "Why is there such universal disagreement?"

First, let me tell you that disagreement is *not universal.* It is largely limited to the United States, and perhaps, Canada. In Europe, virtually all the health authorities – both nutritionists and health-oriented doctors, as well as lay health enthusiasts – agree 100% on all the major health topics. Naturally some minor differences may exist in some areas, but generally there is agreement on all the major issues of nutrition. For instance, in European health food stores, just as in America, you can see shelves full of books on various subjects of nutrition, but you will not find a single one that will recommend heavy meat eating as a health-promoting practice – unless, of course, it is a translated book by an American author! Or, I have visited several dozen of the most reputable spas and fasting clinics in several European countries, but I couldn't find one that would recommend fasting on plain water, or without enemas. All European fasting experts, including the world's greatest authority on fasting, Dr. Otto Buchinger, Jr., agree that juices, broths, herb teas – and enemas! – during fasting assist healing processes and speed recovery.

Why, then, is there such a thorough disagreement among the *American* authorities on the vital questions of nutrition and health?

I can see four major reasons for this:

1. "Scholastic dogmatism and sentimental prejudice"
2. The almighty dollar – commercialism
3. Lack of dependable research on nutrition
4. Outdated, obsolete information.

Scholastic dogmatism and sentimental prejudice

My friend, Dr. Ralph Bircher, of Switzerland, once said: "I know of no branch of science more inclined to scholastic dogmatism and sentimental prejudice than nutrition."

It is conceivable that Adam and Eve had more points of disagreement on food and nutrition than the renowned apple. It is reasonable to assume that man has quarreled about food, what to eat and not to eat, as soon as he stepped upon this earth, and continued to do so throughout his long and colorful history .... not only among the laymen, but especially among the enlightened and the learned as well.

"The Father of Medicine", Hippocrates, wrote 2500 years ago in his discourse on nutrition:

> "If among those who had written on the subject 'which mode of living is the most health-promoting' was one who grasped the matter in its whole width, I would be satisfied with the findings, learned from them and used them. Now, although many have written on the subject, none had a really full knowledge of what he was talking about – one had stressed one aspect, the other some other aspect, but none had hit the essence of the subject."

Doesn't this sound like a pretty accurate description of today's general confusion as to "which mode of living is the most health-promoting"? In a supposedly enlightened and scientific age of the twentieth century, we are still not much wiser than in Hippocrates' time. The authorities today still stress "either one aspect or another", and the disagreement on various issues of nutrition is as great as ever.

Why is it so?

Medicine and nutrition are not exact sciences. Medicine is an art more than a science. When any given drug, vitamin or food brings about a *different* reaction in each individual, you can not talk about *exact science.* Scholastic dogmatism in the area of human nutrition, scientifically rigid adherence to a principle or tenet, without taking the varied and changeable human element into consideration, can only result in pseudo-science and confusion.

Moreover, not only is the study material human, but also scientists, nutritionists and health writers are human. They are very *subjective* in their judgments. Many of their conclusions and beliefs are colored by their own likes and dislikes. We all tend to believe and accept what happens to correspond with our own taste and personal preference. Unscientific? Yes, but very human. Even in the exact sciences, we make provision for the human element, but nutrition, as I have said, is not an exact science.

Scholastic dogmatism and subjective prejudice and judgment must be largely responsible for the unbelievable diversity of opinion in regard to the MDR (Minimum Daily Requirement) of many of the most important nutrients. Here are just a few examples:

- *Protein* is the cornerstone of nutrition. Research on proteins has been going on for a century. You would think the science would be able to tell you a definite answer to the question: what is your daily requirement of protein? The authoritative opinions vary between 25 and 250 grams – take your pick!
- *Vitamin C* is one of the best researched and universally used vitamins. How much should you take each day? The authoritative opinions vary between 30 and 3,000 milligrams.
- *Salt* is another highly disputed nutrient. You are told that you need salt every day. Some authorities recommend 10

grams of salt a day for a healthy person. Some others claim that 0.2 grams is sufficient to satisfy your actual daily need!

The diversity of opinion in regard to the need of many other nutrients is just as great. Why? Again, the subjective judgment, and the difficulty in making an exact scientific conclusion on such a varied research material as human beings.

The almighty dollar – commercialism

A good friend of mine, a fine humanitarian, idealist, and shrewd student of human nature, T. O. McCoye, said: "When the dollar sign enters the field of health or religion, the sincerity and the love fade away." How true!

Americans are the most commercially-minded people in the world. Profit making, or monetary gain, is considered the most important value and goal in virtually every field of human endeavor. Health *business* is no exception. Virtually all health writers, lecturers, and health magazine publishers are ***in business.*** They are trying to *sell* something. For instance, how many lecturers have you heard that didn't have some pills or other products to sell? Also, many health writers produce and sell vitamins, supplements or other products they so highly recommend. *Are you naïve enough to believe that such lecturers and writers can be totally objective in their recommendations?* Or take nutrition magazine publishers. Whatever their personal convictions, they are faced with a choice of either publishing a radical magazine that will condemn as detrimental to health the things man loves to eat most, such as meat, for instance, and sell 5,000 copies per month – or to let the reader have his fat steaks with trimmings, and sell 500,000 copies per month. Indeed, a difficult choice to make for those who look upon their involvement with health and nutrition as *business.*

The lack of dependable research on nutrition

There is virtually no independent nutrition research in the United States. Almost all research is done and/or sponsored by the commercial food industries involved. The giant, multi-billion dollar food processing, chemical and drug industries finance most of nutrition research in the United States, both in private research centers and in the form of grants to the various universities.

For example, the Nutrition Department of one of our leading universities, Harvard, is lavishly financed by America's largest food processors and chemical and drug companies. It is said that "He who pays the piper, calls the tune". It would be naïve to expect that the research, paid for by these producers of processed, devitalized and foodless supermarket foods, would reveal and condemn the real threat to the health of Americans: the processed, devitalized and foodless supermarket foods!

When scientific research is influenced by commercial interests, the average layman is left wallowing in his own ignorance and confusion.

- One day he reads in the paper the statement issued by a certain researcher that tobacco causes cancer; and the next day comes the statement by another researcher that "There is no conclusive evidence . . . "
- One day he reads that fluoridation of the water is harmful to his health; the next day that it is nothing but beneficial.
- One nutritionist writes that processing of foods destroys vital nutrients and contributes to nutritional deficiency diseases; then another claims that modern processed foods are a big boon to health.
- One authority tells him that poisonous residues from pesticides in his foods are harming him in many ways and may be contributing causes to many diseases, including cancer; and in a few days he reads that insecticides are completely harmless to humans.

It all depends on who paid for the research!

As a result, you can find "scientific" evidence and actual research to support *any theory or view* that happens to appeal to you. Nutrition being a very personal matter, where individual preferences, tastes and likes or dislikes play a considerable role, *you can find enough "scientific evidence" to prove any point you want.* If a certain health writer happens to like meat, he can find mountains of scientific evidence to support his high-animal-protein belief. If he happens to be a dye-hard vegetarian, he can find equally impressive evidence to prove his point.

Outdated, obsolete information

The science of nutrition is a relatively new science. Although doctors even before Hippocrates were aware that nutrition plays a major role as causative and corrective factors in disease, they had no scientific means of knowing exactly why it was so. Most of the separate nutritive factors present in foods were isolated only during the last few decades. The scientific methods of analysis of various chemical and organic substances in foods were not perfected until very recently. However, even now, the analytical methods are incomplete. New, hitherto unknown substances in foods are discovered frequently. Just recently, a Finnish researcher discovered 14 new substances in raw onions, hitherto unknown to science.

It has been said that in the last 20 years we have learned more about nutrition than we have learned in the preceding 2000 years. Particularly in the last decade we have experienced an enormous increase in knowledge in many vital areas of nutrition and its effects on man's health. In various research centers of the world, particularly in Germany, Sweden and Russia, nutrition research is done today at an accelerated speed.

- Russians have a government-operated Nutrition Research Institute where extensive research is done on vitamins and their uses and applications in health and disease.
- Russians also study extensively balnealogy (the science of the therapeutic bathing) and curortology (the science of the effects of relaxation, diet and physical fitness on health).
- The Max Plank Institute for Nutritional Research in Germany is making revolutionary discoveries on proteins,

nullifying most of the previous theories and myths scientists have had about proteins.

- The world-famous Karolinska Institute in Stockholm, one of the leading research centers in the world, has been conducting extensive studies for outlining a diet, or nutritional program, that will be most conducive to good health and long life.
- The Swedes also are pioneers in research on fasting, where fasting is done on a mass-scale under controlled conditions.
- The International Society for Research on Nutrition and Diseases of Civilization, with headquarters in Germany, is busily engaged in extensive research and compilation of all available data on nutrition and its relation to health.

All the above sources of reliable scientific information are new, not available just a few short years ago. Nutrition research is growing so fast that those who are not engaged fulltime in following what is happening are left behind, repeating over and over the old, outdated and antiquated ideas and theories, many of which have long been disproved. *The health books written ten years ago or earlier, are largely obsolete as far as reliable nutrition information is concerned.*

This is one reason for such wide disagreement and confusion among health writers and lecturers in the United States. Most of the health authorities are not following the recent developments in international nutrition research. Most of the lecturers have never heard of the independent research sources I enumerated a few paragraphs back. Many of the American health writers, some of the most popular ones, wrote their books one, two or three decades ago. Their conclusions are based on outdated and insufficient data. Some popular writers use American medical journals as major sources of nutritional information. Knowing how most American research, sponsored by food-processing industries, is done, this source of information would be the least reliable of all.

I am mindful of the great responsibility that goes with the ambitious project of writing this *ARE YOU CONFUSED?* book. I have decided to write it for two reasons: *First,* the great confusion among the honest health-seekers I constantly meet; and, *second,* my humble conviction that by doing constant, full-time research for the last 20 years and keeping abreast of all the latest scientific developments in the field of nutrition, I have the needed information and knowledge that can be helpful in straightening out some of the most common myths, fallacies, misconceptions and half-truths relative to nutrition and health.

May I add here that I do not wish to condemn or criticize writers, lecturers, or publishers individually or collectively. I am sure that most health writers are sincere, and much of their advice is helpful and has been beneficial to many a reader. Although by the very nature of this work I will have to point out misconceptions and errors in various writings and teachings, this should not be construed as a personal attack or criticism. The purpose of this book is not a negative fault-finding, but a constructive, positive attempt to help both the students and the teachers with information on the latest facts. Anyone who has read more than three health books by American health writers knows by personal experience that this *De-CONFUSION Book* is needed, indeed – and needed badly.

The difficult position of the nutrition advisor

There is another point to consider. When a "health expert", writer or lecturer assumes the role of an authority, teacher and leader – and acquires a large following of disciples or "students" – his position on various health issues will often become fixed and, thus, open-minded, objective judgement made impossible. Imagine a hypothetical writer who, several decades ago, wrote several books which promulgated the high-protein myth. He is practically compelled to cling to that view the rest of his life, even if he personally became convinced through research that his original theories were erroneous. What would his millions of readers and students think if, after advising a high-protein diet for decades, he would suddenly change his views? He has to defend his teachings with every possible "scientific support", totally ignoring the more impressive scientific support which proves that his former position was wrong. It takes a great man to admit a mistake and change his mind.

To sum up this chapter: With such thorough confusion and disagreement among the authorities on vital questions of nutrition and health; with scholastic dogmatism and reliance on outdated information; with the lack of independent nutrition research in the United States; with the ever-present commercial profit-motive entering the health field and confusing the issues – *is it any wonder that the honest health-seeker is left wallowing in his own ignorance, lost in a confusing labyrinth of contradictory claims?*

Chapter 2

High or Low Protein Diet– Which Is Better?

This is the most controversial question among American health authorities and health-conscious people. No other issue of nutrition is affected more by personal likes and habits than the issue of animal proteins. Many of America's most respected health writers have recommended a high-protein diet as a must for optimum health. During my lectures the question of proteins brings the most heated arguments.

A high protein requirement is the absolute must of any "respectable" American health system. We are so brainwashed by this "high protein-low carbohydrate" myth that even a mere suggestion of possible erroneousness of this premise would jeopardize one's credibility. Yet, practically all of Who's Who in the European health field are unanimous in their endorsement of a *low protein diet,* particularly *low animal protein diet,* as the diet most conducive to good health and long life. The empirical evidence in support of the low protein diet is equally impressive.

Why the high-protein craze?

The scientific fact that your body is made mostly of proteins may be largely responsible for the high-protein myth. It is true, of course, that proteins are vital nutritive elements and are absolutely necessary in your nutrition. But the present recommendation of "lots" of protein in the diet is based on antiquated research of the 19th century. Most of the advocates of the high-protein diet repeat in a parrot-like fashion the erroneous conclusions made by the 19th century German researchers Von Liebig, Von Voit, and Max Rubner. These scientists came to the conclusion that man's minimum daily requirement of protein was 120 grams. Although these conclusions were based on very primitive and unscientifically conducted research – where, for example, no distinction was made between animal and vegetable protein, or between raw and cooked protein – much of today's argument for a high protein intake is based on the calculations of these German scientists. Nutrition courses in our universities and medical schools today are teaching the protein requirement tables made by these 19th century men. This in spite of the fact that the latest research from various parts of the world shows that our actual protein need is far below that which it was previously believed to be.

Of course, the commercial motive even here has played a decisive role in building up the high-protein cult. There are huge economic interests – the multibillion dollar livestock, dairy and meat-packing industry – involved in promoting the high-protein diet. These industries sponsor most of the protein research. And through the powerful advertising in every media, including the "Beef for Health" stickers on automobile bumpers, they see to it that you never forget that you need "lots of protein" for health. We have been brainwashed by the high protein propaganda from every possible direction for half a century.

How much protein do you actually need?

During the last few decades, a growing number of independent researchers have been showing that our present beliefs in regard to protein are outdated and that the actual daily need for protein in human nutrition is far below that which has long been considered necessary.

World-famous Swedish nutritionist, Dr. Ragnar Berg, whose works on nutrition are used as text books in many medical schools, made an extensive research on protein and concluded that 30 grams of protein in the daily diet is a generous allowance.

Finnish scientist, Dr. V. O. Sivén, arrived at the exact same amount – 30 grams. American scientist, Dr. R. Chittenden, found, in his extensive experiments with athletes and soldiers, that 30 to 50 grams of protein a day is sufficient for maximum physical performance. He also demonstrated that physical performance in sports and heavy physical work *is better on a low protein diet.* Dr. D. M. Hegsted, of Harvard University, found that 27 grams a day is the average person's daily need for protein. And research made by Dr. William C. Rose has shown that only 20 grams a day of mixed proteins (of which only about 2/3 are so-called complete) is sufficient for our needs. The recent studies by German Professor, Dr. K. Eimer, showed that athletes' performance improved after they switched from a 100 gram-a-day animal protein diet to a 50 gram-a-day vegetable protein diet. And, finally, recently a Japanese researcher, Dr. Kuratsune, showed that 25-30 grams of protein a day is sufficient to sustain good health.

Based on all this recent research, and taking into consideration great variation in the protein need of each individual, the generous conclusions would be that 40 to 50 grams a day of protein, up to 2/3 derived from vegetable sources, is sufficient for optimum health.

Can you get too much protein?

Yes, indeed. You can get too much of fat and carbohydrates, although they are essential nutrients. Even too much of certain vitamins or minerals is harmful and may cause ill health. And so it is also with proteins. As essential and important as they are, too much protein in the diet, especially cooked animal protein, can cause serious health disorders.

Proteins in excess of actual need can not be stored by the body, and are only burned as a fuel for energy. As an energy food, however, proteins are inferior to carbohydrates or fats. The digestion of proteins in excess of the actual need leaves toxic residues of metabolic waste products, which contribute to self-intoxication and consequent disease.

Here is a partial list of what too much protein in your diet can cause:

- Toxic residues in the tissues. Professor Kofranyi, of famous Max Plank Institute for Nutritional Research, said, "More protein than needed builds only more toxins."
- Biochemical imbalance in tissues and resultant over-acidity.
- Accumulation of uric acid, urea and toxic purines in the tissues.
- Diminished strength and endurance. Drs. Chittenden and Fisher concluded that uric acid, urea, and purines of meat poison and interfere with muscle and nerve function.
- Intestinal putrefaction and resultant constipation and auto-toxemia.
- Vitamin B_6 deficiency.
- Arteriosclerosis, heart disease and kidney damage.
- Arthritis. Recently, Dr. Gerber, professor at New York University, said that "faulty protein metabolism" may be one of the contributing causes of arthritis.

A good rule to follow in regard to protein is: enough but not too much.

Meat protein versus vegetable protein

You have been told that "you need animal proteins for optimum health." You also have been told that "only animal proteins are complete, and vegetable proteins are incomplete." Both statements are false. Again, in all probability they are based on antiquated research. Dr. Thomas, in 1909, coined the term *biological value of protein.* Proteins are made of amino acids. Of 20 or so amino acids, eight are considered *essential.* That is, they can not be produced within the body and must be supplied by the food you eat. Not all foods contain all the amino acids. Foods which contain all the essential amino acids are called the *complete protein foods.* Those which lack one or more of the essential amino acids are called the *incomplete protein foods.*

Until very recently it has been assumed that only animal proteins – meat, fish, eggs and milk – contained complete proteins, and that all vegetable proteins were incomplete. Recent research has proven this assumption to be erroneous. Research from one of the leading institutions for nutritional research in the world, the Max Plank Institute in Germany, showed that many vegetables, fruits, seeds, nuts and grains are excellent sources of complete proteins. This is corroborated by research from many other research centers. Soybeans, sunflower seeds, sesame seeds, almonds, potatoes, and most fruits and green vegetables contain complete proteins. Furthermore, recent research has established two extremely important facts, hitherto unknown to science:

1. *Vegetable proteins are higher in biological value than animal proteins.* For example, proteins in potatoes are biologically superior to proteins in meat, eggs or milk.

2. *Raw proteins have higher biological value than cooked proteins.* You need only one-half the amount of proteins if you eat raw vegetable proteins instead of cooked animal proteins.

Potatoes, a stepchild of American nutrition, are actually excellent health food and a good source of superior quality proteins. In Germany, ten per cent of the average dietary intake of protein is obtained from potatoes. It has been demonstrated that people have lived on potatoes as the sole source of proteins as long as six years and enjoyed excellent health. All green vegetables have complete proteins of highest biological value.

"Where do you get your proteins?"

This is the most frequently asked question by heavy meat-eaters as soon as they find out that I do not advise meat eating.

Did you ever wonder where the wild horse, who builds a magnificent body in a couple of years, gets all his proteins? From the grass he eats, of course. And where do about one half of the world's population, who do not eat meat for religious or other reasons, get their proteins?

The answer is that our Creator in his wisdom, knowing how important proteins are for man and animal, made them a part of every *naturally occuring food.* Every plant, every vegetable, every fruit and every seed contains some protein. *It is virtually impossible not to get enough protein in your diet provided you have enough to eat of natural, unrefined foods.* The proponents of a high protein meat diet often refer to the big-bellied, starved African children as an example of protein deficiency. These children suffer from protein deficiency not because they eat a protein-deficient diet, but because they are *starving.* The diet of raw vegetables, fruits, seeds, grains, and nuts plus milk and cheese – so-called lacto-vegetarian diet, as described in the next chapter – will supply in abundance not only all the proteins you need but also with all the other nutritive substances, such as vitamins, minerals, carbohydrates, fatty acids, enzymes and trace elements.

Let me re-emphasize that the proteins in vegetables, fruits and many seeds and nuts are biologically superior to animal proteins. And your protein needs can be satisfied by one half the amount of proteins if you eat them raw instead of cooked.

Common fallacies about protein

You have been told that *"you need lots of protein each day."* This is a typical example of half-truth. It is true that your body needs proteins each day for its vital functions and new-building of cells. But you don't have to *eat* proteins each day. Your body can exist without any food, and consequently without any proteins, for weeks and months, as evidenced by prolonged therapeutic fasting. It is a general observation that the protein level of the blood (serum albumin reading) of fasting patients remains constant and normal during the whole fasting period, *in spite of the fact that no protein is consumed.* The reason for this is that the proteins in your body are in the so-called dynamic state: they are constantly changed from one form to another, being decomposed and resynthesized from blood plasma amino acids. Amino acids from the old and broken-down cells are not wasted, but are re-used for the building of new cells. Thus the body is using and re-using the same proteins again and again where they are needed. This shows that you don't have to eat high-protein meals every day, although your body does need protein every day.

Another common misconception about protein is that "*only complete proteins can satisfy your protein needs.*" It is a well established physiological fact that foods with so-called incomplete proteins will complement one another, *rendering their total available protein content biologically complete.* Tortillas and beans, or a whole-wheat bread and cheese sandwich are good examples. Corn, wheat or beans are, seperately, incomplete protein foods, but eaten in the above combinations the proteins become complete.

Are meat eaters healthier than vegetarians?

Some popular health writers (who apparently would rather be popular than truthful) tell you that lots of animal protein is a must for optimum health.

They will tell you that meat eaters are healthier than vegetarians. Haven't they ever met Seventh-Day Adventists? There are a million of them, mostly living right here in the United States. Seventh-Day Adventists supply grand-scale scientific evidence supporting the low-animal protein diet.

A recent study conducted by several medical doctors, show that Seventh-Day Adventists, who do not eat meat for religious reasons, have:

- 40% less coronary disease
- 400% less death rate from respiratory diseases
- 100% lower mortality rate from all causes
- 1000% lower death rate from lung cancer
- 50% less dental caries among their children

These statistics speak for themselves. They repudiate clearly the myth perpetrated by the meat-eating propagandists that meat eaters are healthier than vegetarians. The above is an extraordinarily remarkable scientific study made by reputable medical men and reported in the Journal of the American Medical Association which shows that a large group of people, who live in the United States under seemingly the same conditions as the rest of us, *but do not eat meat,* have such superior health compared to the rest of the Americans!

There is no better way than the *empirical* way to prove any nutritional theory. If one can put the theory into practice or see what results it has produced through the centuries, even milleniums, of actual application – then it is worth more than bookshelves of scientific reasoning and laboratory proofs.

Such empirical evidence of the superiority of low animal protein diet is easily available. Here are a few convincing facts:

1. The *Hunza* people, living in an isolated kingdom in the Himalayas, are considered "the healthiest people in the world" by all researchers who studied their health condition, including, famous British physician Dr. R. McCarrison, who lived among them for years. Cancer, heart disease, diabetes, rheumatic diseases, high blood pressure, arteriosclerosis, arthritis and many other diseases common to western countries, are unknown in Hunza. Their longevity and endurance are legendary. They live up to 90 and 100 and are virile, strong and active after they reach 80 and 90. All researchers who studied them agree that their diet is the major factor in their unusual health and longevity. The Hunza diet is a *high natural carbohydrate-low animal protein diet!* Their staples are grains, such as wheat, barley, buckwheat; fruits, mostly apricots, apples and grapes; assorted vegetables, eaten mostly raw; and very little milk,

mostly goat milk. They eat few eggs, and very little meat, only on festive occasions, not more often than once a month.

2. In the last few years, researchers discovered two primitive tribes, in different parts of the world, who lived in total isolation from the civilized world for more than a thousand years. One was a Yemenite tribe of Semitic origin; the other, Maya Indians of Yucatan. Scientists who studied these people were amazed at their phenomenal health condition, long life and freedom from diseases. They also discovered that the diet of these primitive people with superior health was a *low animal protein-high natural carbohydrate diet!* Yemenites ate meat occasionally and sparingly, but the Maya Indians were 100% vegetarians, their main food being corn, beans, and vegetables.

3. *Russians* are known for their good health, longevity and endurance. They have seven times more centenarians per million than the United States. *They are low protein people.* 78.5% of their protein need is derived from vegetable sources, and only 21.5% from animal sources. (In the U.S., 29% is vegetable and 71% is animal protein!) Futhermore, a suprisingly great number of Russia's 21,000 centenarians are total vegetarians! Russia's health records are far better than America's. Their mortality rate is 7.3 per thousand as compared to 9.4 in the United-States. The life expectancy of the Russian male is 70.1 – the American male's is only 66.7 years.

4. *Bulgarians* are among the healthiest peoples in Europe. They are the tallest people in south Europe and they possess great vitality and longevity. There are more centenarians in Bulgaria than in any other country in the world – 1,600 persons, 100 years or over, per million of population, as compared to only 9 persons per million among heavy meat-eating Americans. Bulgarians eat very little meat. Their diet consists largely of black bread (most whole rye and barley), vegetables and soured milk in the form of yogurt and kefir. One study made by a Swedish doctor showed that of 158 Bulgarians, 100 years or over, only 5 ate meat regularly.

High or low?

The scientific and empirical evidence presented in this chapter clearly shows that the diet most conducive to optimum health and long life is not the *high protein,* but the *high natural carbohydrate-low animal protein,* diet. Americans eat more meat and more proteins than most other nations in the world. Americans also lead the world in cancer, heart disease, arthritis, obesity, high blood pressure, multiple sclerosis, mortality rate, miscarriages and birth deformities, and other degenerative diseases. Heart disease is our greatest killer. By the way, studies have shown that a low protein vegetarian diet can prevent 97% of coronary occlusions, or heart disease.

This presentation should, however, not be misconstrued to imply that you should minimize the importance of protein in your diet. You need, to be sure, good protein in sufficient amounts for the proper functioning of all your organs, and for the maintenance of good health. But because proteins are so important it does not automatically follow that you can eat unrestricted amounts of them.

Low animal protein-high natural carbohydrate diet holds the greatest potential for optimum health, prevention of disease, greater vitality and extended longevity.

This is not a theory, hypothesis or wishful thinking, but a firmly established scientific conclusion, based on the latest research and empirical facts.

In the next chapter you will learn how to plan your low animal protein meals in the context of your complete nutrition program for optimum health.

Chapter 3

What Is the True Macrobiotic Diet ?

One of the most hopeful and positive attributes of our much discussed youth is their intense interest in health and nutrition. Why they revolt, burn buildings, use drugs, protest government actions or seem to behave antisocially at times, would be outside the context of this book to discuss. But since such a large percentage of American youth is "awakened" to the perils of the devitalized American foods and shows such an extraordinary interest in better nutrition, it is fitting to help these youth to the proper orientation in this confusing field.

It is significant that it took a man from the East to awaken the interest of American youth in health-building nutrition. Disillusioned in the Western, materialistically-geared, demoralized way of life and in the failure of the Western religions to protect and preserve the high life-values, the American youth have been looking toward the East for answers. Therefore, what the dynamic American health-prophets were unable to do – to reach the hearts of the youth – the soft-spoken Japanese, Dr. Georges Ohsawa, achieved. The only problem is that the Macrobiotic diet, which has so fascinated many young people, *is not what it is purported to be,* and many of those who have looked to it and hoped that it would improve their health, have been sadly disappointed.

What are macrobiotics?

Those who think that macrobiotics were invented by Dr. Ohsawa may be surprised to know that the origin of macrobiotics goes back 150 years to a great physician, researcher and professor, Christopher Wilhelm Hufeland, who lived and worked in Berlin. He wrote a book which he called *MAKROBIOTIK – THE ART OF PROLONGING HUMAN LIFE.* Ohsawa merely borrowed the word originated by Hufeland and built his own dietary system around it, giving it an oriental touch.

Originally, macrobiotics meant "the art of living longer." But the prospect of a long life is attractive only if it means a life of vibrant health, free from disease. With the advance of the modern chemical and technological age, the environmental health-destroying factors are making the art of living in good health more and more difficult with every passing day. The Sword of Damocles – the environment-caused diseases of civilization – is hanging over us and is threatening our very existence. The harmony between man and his environment is broken. Man has become his own worst enemy. He has poisoned his planet, air, water, and soil. He has devitalized, denatured and poisoned his own food supply. Our civilization can appropriately be called the age of chemical orgy. By the indiscriminate use of chemicals in his total environment, man has brought upon himself a host of environment-induced diseases, rightly called the *diseases of civilization.* Cancer, heart disease, arthritis, diabetes, arteriosclerosis, emphysema, high blood pressure – these are typical examples of man's self-induced ills, or diseases of civilization. The gradual deterioration of health has now reached catastrophic proportions. More than half of America's adult population is chronically ill.

Macrobiotics, therefore, must have a broader meaning than just an "art of living longer", in order to be useful for the twentieth century man during the last decades of this civilization. Today's definition of macrobiotics is:

- The art of living longer in good health and freedom from disease.
- The art of living in a denatured, adulterated and poisoned environment.
- The art of preventing premature aging and living *younger* longer.

The difficult art of macrobiotics

To achieve this goal – a long life of youthful vitality and freedom from disease – is becoming more difficult every year, as health-destroying factors in man's environment are multiplying at a faster and faster speed.

Although the situation is precarious and at times seems hopeless – as if man has already reached the point of no return in his senseless drive toward self-destruction – our self-preservation instinct tells us not to give up, to continue trying to change the tide for the better. The tragedy of the whole situation is that most people do not realize the seriousness, or even the existence, of the real danger. They still live under the delusion that the great progress of technological, chemical, medical and pharmacological science is improving the quality of life, extending the life expectancy, eliminating diseases, and bringing them nothing but an easier and happier life. That's what science has been promising them, and that's what they think they are still going to get. This dream could have been realized, except for the one thing which the dreamers of scientific utopia forgot to take into consideration – *man's greed.* It is man's greed that has turned the potential of science into his Sword of Damocles.

Those of us who are aware of what's going on, *what can we do* to protect ourselves from the health-threatening dangers of man's denatured environment? Can we still live healthy lives and prevent disease and premature aging?

It must be admitted that it is not easy, but it can be done. The best way to start is with your nutrition.

Nutrition – the number one factor in macrobiotics

"Which is worse, smoking or drinking?" a famed health lecturer was once asked. His classical answer reflects the message of this book:

"Neither one is as bad as malnutrition."

Nutrition is singularly the most important factor affecting one's health. There are other factors, of course: smoking, drinking, severe mental and emotional stress, lack of sleep and relaxation, insufficient exercise, etc. But none of these can bring about such rapid and devastating deterioration of health as faulty nutrition, or malnutrition can.

If faulty nutrition can destroy one's health, then it would be logical to conclude that proper or improved nutrition would be the most important factor in preventing disease or restoring one's health.

"Our food must be our medicine – our medicine must be our food", said Hippocrates. The question is: *which* food is our medicine? I guess that in Hippocrates time, 2,500 years ago, most any food was medicine. But much that goes under the name of food today is closer to suicidal poison than to the health-restoring medicine.

On the basis of existing scientific and empirical evidence, and the latest findings of the International Society for Research on Nutrition and the Diseases of Civilization, the macrobiotic program of vital nutrition with greatest potential for optimum health, maximum vitality, long life and prevention of disease, should comply with the following rules.

THE SEVEN BASIC RULES OF SCIENTIFIC VITALIZING NUTRITION FOR OPTIMUM HEALTH AND LONG LIFE

1. EAT ONLY NATURAL FOODS

Your body is a living organism, a part of a complex universe and subject to the laws of nature. It *must* be nourished by natural, organic food elements in their natural, unaltered state in order to survive and function in good health.

What are *natural* foods? Foods grown on fertile soil under natural conditions, and consumed in their natural state are *natural foods.* Foods grown in depleted soils with the help of chemicals and processed by heat, irradiation or chemical treatment, are *not natural* foods.

Here are some examples:

Eggs laid by hens running outdoors in sunlight and eating grass, seeds, insects and worms – and in the company of roosters! – are natural, fertile eggs, with dark yolks and full, nutritional value. But eggs produced by "cooped-up" chickens in an "egg factory", by hens who never see daylight or rooster and are fed only synthetic medicated mash, are *not natural* eggs. Such eggs are infertile, they will not produce chickens, their yolks are pale, their chemical composition is altered, their vitamin content is lower and their total nutritional value is way below that of a natural egg. Among other things, eggs produced by cooped-up chickens contain twice as much saturated fats as the natural eggs do. Such eggs can not possibly sustain the health of those who eat them.

Natural, raw, unpasteurized milk has more vitamins and enzymes; the proteins and minerals of such milk are easily digested and assimilated by the body. Pasteurization reduces the vitamin and enzyme content and makes minerals, fatty acids and proteins less assimilable and digestible.

Natural fruits, vegetables and grains should grow in healthy, humus-rich soils, without chemical fertilizers or toxic sprays. Natural foods contain more protein, more vitamins, more minerals and other nutrients, particularly the vital enzymes, than the canned or packaged, unnatural or processed foods bought at your supermarket.

It should be kept in mind that our knowledge of food composition is very incomplete. Scientists who tried to feed test animals a synthetic diet composed of *all* the nutritive substances known to science, have found that animals could live in seemingly good health, and even have reproductive capacity. However, from the second and third generation, animals lost their power to reproduce and the whole strain gradually died. Also, their health condition and the growth rate were adversely affected by the synthetic diet. These experiments prove that natural foods contain more than just all the known or discovered nutrients. When you eat natural, unprocessed and unadulterated foods, you will get the benefit of all these undiscovered, but vital, substances as well.

That your health and your longevity are in a direct relationship to the *naturalness* of the foods you eat is a well-established scientific fact. Dr. Weston A. Price, Vilhjalmur Steffansson, Dr. McCarrison, Arnold DeVries, and many others, who made extensive travels and studies of diet habits and their relation to health and longevity of practically every "primitive" people in the world, have found that when the diet was made of natural, fresh, unprocessed foods, grown in their own environment, the people had no disease or tooth decay. Conversely, where they discovered people subject to dental decay and various other degenerative diseases of civilized man, they invariably found that they ate denatured, cooked, processed foods, and that white flour, canned foods, and white sugar had made their way to them from more "civilized" countries.

Moreover, regardless of the composition of the diet – whether it was exclusively vegetarian, lacto-vegetarian, predominantly meat or largely dairy-product diet – as long as the foods were *natural,* unprocessed, and largely eaten raw, the people maintained vibrant health, lived long, and enjoyed youthful vitality.

Arnold DeVries has studied the historical records of the North and South American Indians, Eskimos, Asians, Africans, Australian aborigines, New Zealand Maories, and people living on Pacific and Atlantic islands, and found that all of them enjoyed glowing health, great fertility and almost incredible endurance. Diseases were almost unknown. Women had fast and painless childbirths, and were usually back to their work in the fields an hour later. Men could run all day without fatigue. There was no tooth decay, or loss of sight or hearing, or gray hair. Although statistical life expectancy was low because of the poor sanitation, most of those who survived lived to be 100 years or over. DeVries also found that as soon as "civilized" foods were introduced to these people, their health began to decline. Childbirth became painful and prolonged; tooth decay made its impact; vitality and endurance abated; and they gradually became subject to all the diseases of "civilized" people.

Synthetic, denatured, altered and devitalized foods will not sustain health, but will inevitably bring about a degeneration of normal bodily functions and ultimately disease and premature aging.

2. EAT ONLY WHOLE FOODS

Whole foods are simply foods which still contain all the nutrients nature has put into them – not less and not more! – complete, unfragmented, unrefined, neither fortified nor enriched. Whole wheat bread, potatoes in jackets, brown rice, sugar cane, oranges – are whole foods. White bread, instant potatoes, polished rice, white sugar and orange juice – are not whole foods. They are fragmented, concentrated or refined foods from which important nutrient factors have been processed out, destroyed, or removed. More than 90% of all the foods on the average American table today have been tampered with in one way or another, and most of the vital nutrients have been either taken out of them or destroyed.

Breakfast cereals, processed oils, fruit juices, all products made with white sugar and white flour are typical examples of such fragmented, devitalized and adulterated foods. Every time a natural substance is removed from a food, the natural balance is disturbed. Every time a chemical is added to the food, the natural balance is also disturbed. Every time food is refined or fragmented, such as extracting sugar from sugar cane or sugar beets, or separating the wheat endosperm (from which wheat flour is made) from the whole wheat kernel – the natural balance is disturbed. When you eat such fragmented foods, they disturb the normal bio-chemical and metabolic processes within your body. It took thousands of years for your body to adjust its bio-chemical processes to the composition of natural foods. When suddenly the composition of foods is altered, your body is not able to re-adjust its chemical processes. This causes havoc in the body chemistry with disease as the ultimate result.

The two worst examples of fragmented foods are white sugar and white flour – these two nutritionless monstrosities, disguised under the name of food, are responsible more than anything else for the deterioration of health in civilized countries. During World War II, in European countries, the consumption of white flour and white sugar was sharply reduced due to rationing. The statistics also showed a sharp reduction in the incidence of many degenerative diseases during these years, notably a sharp decrease in diabetes. Note, that although the use of *refined carbohydrates* decreased, the consumption of *whole, natural carbohydrates,* such as whole grains, actually increased during the war. This proves that natural, whole carbohydrate foods are health-promoting, whereas refined carbohydrates are detrimental to health.

Whole wheat, for example, is a good source of vitamin E. But it would take more than 200 slices of white bread to secure a proper daily requirement of this vital vitamin, because most of it has been removed with the wheat germ in processing. The same goes with the B-vitamins, minerals, best proteins and the natural oils of the wheat. If you eat *enriched* bread, do not think you get these nutrients anyway, since they allegedly have been added to the bread. None of the vitamin E, oils, minerals, or proteins have been added; and from more than 15 vitamins of the B-complex that have been removed in processing, only 3 have been returned in insignificant amounts. *If this is enrichment, I'd like to know what is impoverishment!*

The American housewife, brainwashed by T.V. commercials, feeds her family "enriched" white bread, believing that it will help to build "stronger bodies in ten different ways". But in the refining process, the white bread has lost 65 to 75% of all the important natural vitamins and minerals, and only a few of them have been replaced with inorganic, synthetic chemical vitamins that lack the nutritional resemblance to the organic life-factors that were removed. One nutritionist said that such "enrichment" is similar to robbing a man of his wallet, watch and glasses, and giving him a bus token to get home on! Because vitamins are synergistic in their action, when part of a complex, such as one or more B-vitamins, has been removed, serious deficiencies are likely to arise. Enrichment may actually do more harm than good.

The value of whole, unrefined foods was dramatically demonstrated on a grand scale during the First World War. Denmark was plagued by a serious food shortage. The government assigned Dr. M. Hindhede, the director of the Danish Institute of Nutrition Research, to design a program for protecting the nation from the hunger threat. The first action of Hindhede was to increase the whole-grain production by limiting the livestock production and curtailing the sale of meat, and thus saving grain for human consumption. Production of alcoholic beverages was banned for the same reason. Also, grain processing was stopped and only whole-grain bread and cereals were allowed to be sold. Farmers were directed and encouraged to produce more grain, green vegetables, fruits, milk and butter, instead of meat.

These simple, but from a nutritional standpoint revolutionary changes in eating habits, resulted in spectacular and rapid changes in the health condition of the whole nation. The death rate dropped over 40% in one year. Diseases that affected other European countries, including the dreaded influenza epidemic, by-passed Denmark. In only a few years, Denmark became the healthiest nation in all of Europe!

In those regions of India where polished white rice is the staple food, the incidence of diabetes and peptic ulcers is much higher than in the other regions, such as Punjab, where instead of rice the dietary staples are coarse wheat and corn.

In Africa, where natives eat large quantities of sugar cane, there is virtually no diabetes or dental caries. When these natives, however, move to the cities and begin to eat white sugar, they rapidly develop caries, diabetes, ulcers and other diseases of civilization. Dr. John Yudkin, of London University, has conclusively demonstrated that white sugar and white flour products are the major cause of heart disease.

Whole foods are an absolute must for optimum health. Whole foods contain not only *complete nutrition,* but also all the enzymes and other factors necessary for the proper, effective digestion and good assimilation of each particular food. When some of the vitamins, minerals and enzymes are removed, as in the case of white sugar or white flour, as well as other refined or processed foods, the digestion and assimilation is incomplete – with nutritional deficiencies and disease as the ultimate result.

3. EAT ONLY LIVING FOODS

Dr. Robert Bell hit the nail on the head when he said, "Man is the only creature upon this earth who spoils his food before he eats it." Man's slow degeneration to the present inferno of diseases started with the discovery of cooking. Since then man seems to have been using his creative imagination and unlimited inventiveness for devising newer and newer means of ruining the nutritional value of his food. The latest of these devices is irradiation. Now you can buy potatoes, yams, onions, and other vegetables that do not sprout and will keep "fresh" forever. What this irradiation with atomic rays does to the life-sustaining power of the food nobody really knows, as yet. The only thing the processors are concerned about is, of course, the marketing convenience and the longer shelf life.

Cooking destroys enzymes 100%. Enzymes are vital catalysts, absolutely essential for the proper digestion and assimilation of the food, as well as for all other functions in your body. Nobel Prize Winner, Professor Virtanen, from Finland, has demonstrated that in the process of chewing raw foods, new active substances are formed in the mouth with the help of enzymes. It is estimated that about 600 various enzymes are essential for human health, but all enzymes in foods are destroyed in cooking. In addition, cooking destroys many of the vitamins. Water-soluble vitamins B and C are particularly vulnerable to the effect of heat and cooking. Minerals also are depleted by cooking and are usually thrown away with the cooking water.

Prolonged storage, freezing, drying, salting and canning, are all more or less destructive to the nutritional value of the food. Fresh vegetables stored at room temperature for only one day lose up to 50 per cent of their vitamin C. Blanching and freezing destroys vitamins B_1 and B_2. Since the average American diet consists up to 90 per cent of cooked, frozen or otherwise processed foods, it is no wonder that half of the population is suffering from various degrees of vitamin deficiencies and malnutrition.

Raw, living foods contain all the nutritive elements in the right proportion and balance. Contrary to the popular notion, most foods in their raw state are easier to digest than the same foods in their cooked state. This is particularly true of all fruits and most vegetables and grains.

Even moderate heating destroys nutritional value of foods. Pasteurization of milk destroys some of the vitamins and all of the enzymes. Lewis J. Silvers, M.D., says that at least three factors in milk are destroyed by the process of pasteurization: an anemia-prevention factor, an ulcer-prevention factor, and an arthritis-prevention factor.

The *therapeutic* value of raw foods is well known. In most European biological clinics raw foods are used in healing of many common diseases, such as cancer, arthritis, multiple sclerosis, etc. The famous Gerson cure for cancer is based primarily on raw foods and raw juices. In animal tests, arthritis was experimentally caused by feeding animals cooked foods exclusively.

Raw, living foods are equally known for their *prophylactic* (or disease-preventive) value. Furthermore, raw foods act as a cleansing agent on the digestive and eliminative systems and are the best preventive measure agains constipation.

The aging-preventive and rejuvenative property of raw foods was scientifically demonstrated and explained in European and Japanese research. Raw plant foods increase the micro-electric tension in cell tissue, as was discovered by the Viennese scientists investigating cell permeability. Increased micro-electric tension in the cell tissue improves cell oxygenation, stimulates cell metabolism, increases the cell's resistance to aging, speeds the process of cell renewal – in short, improves the cell's metabolism and prevents biochemical suffocation. Japanese researchers at the University of Kyushu have shown that raw plant foods contain substances that help the body in its fight against disease-producing agents.

In terms of application, many would find eating raw foods exclusively too difficult. But you should make an effort to eat fresh, raw foods as much as possible. At least two thirds of all foods eaten should be in their natural, raw state. Practically all fruits and vegetables can be eaten raw. If cooking is absolutely necessary, food should be cooked as little as possible, preferably steamed with little or no water. All broth, of course, should be used also.

Eat all nuts raw. You will discover that they are much tastier and easier to digest in their raw state, than when they are roasted and salted. Many seeds and grains can be eaten raw, especially when they are sprouted.* Raw, unpasteurized milk is available at better health food stores.

Remember, *cooked food is dead food.* Only living foods can build healthy bodies.

4. EAT ONLY POISON-FREE FOODS

I must admit that it is much easier to *give* such advice than to *follow* it in today's poisoned world. Poisons in food are the greatest menace to health today. It is almost impossible to obtain food stuffs that are free from poisonous residues and additives. Fruits and vegetables contain residues of dozens of poisonous pesticides, waxes, bleaches, artificial colorings and preservatives. Meat, milk, butter and poultry contain, in addition to DDT and other insecticides, residues of hormones, antibiotics and other drugs used to speed animal growth. Processed meats, bread, cereals, and canned foods and drinks are loaded with some of the nearly one thousand different chemicals which

---

*See Chapter 16 for Directions.

are now used in the food-processing industry. And many of these have never been tested for their possible toxicity!

There is a growing concern among world scientists that mankind is committing slow suicide by poisoning himself with all these foreign substances in his food and his environment. Many of the newest diseases are directly related to the poisons in our foods. The growing incidence of birth deformities is one of the most conspicuous diseases attributed to the poisonous drugs and residues in foods.

The American public is becoming more and more aware of the dangers of DDT, malathion, parathion, and other pesticides in foods. The beginning of a new decade, the seventies, brought one hope of a nation-wide awakening in regard to the environment. DDT was banned in several states in 1969, and in 1970 the Federal Government took action of restricting DDT use in the whole country. But one of the gravest dangers to our health, of which we only seldom hear, is a gradual but universal lead-poisoning. In Europe, scientists are alarmed at the incredible speed with which lead is poisoning our environment. Lead comes to the atmosphere mostly from the automobiles which burn gasoline treated with lead. It pollutes the air, settles in the soils and is absorbed by the fruits and vegetables. Tests made in Germany show that some of the vegetables, especially carrots, contain deadly amounts of lead. Many poisonings from eating lead-containing carrots were registered. Lead has a degenerative effect on the central nervous system and *affects genetic forces,* as found by Russian scientists. Even in small amounts it causes degenerative changes in the liver, kidneys, heart and other organs.

Every effort, therefore, should be made to obtain poison-free organically grown foods. They are often available in health food stores. If supermarket-quality vegetables are used, they should be washed carefully or peeled. Cucumbers, green and red peppers, tomatoes, celery, carrots, apples, pears, grapes, and cherries can be washed and brushed in warm water with soap or mild detergent, then rinsed well several times and finally rinsed under cold running water to remove the traces of soap.

Remember, just rinsing produce in cold water will do no good; most sprays and waxes are oil-soluble and plain cold water will not remove them at all.

5. EAT HIGH NATURAL CARBOHYDRATE-LOW ANIMAL PROTEIN DIET

You have learned in the previous chapter that the diet with the greatest potential for optimum health and long life is a *high natural carbohydrate-low animal protein diet.* This is contrary to what you have read and heard from present-day nutritionists and "authorities". Even the most respected nutritional advisors and health writers in the United States have been so misled by the high-protein propaganda and by the misleading protein research, sponsored by the meat-packing and dairy industries, that they also fell prey to this high-protein myth. They continue repeating the well-established lie that "we can never get enough protein", This, in spite of the following facts:

- Americans, who eat more protein than any other nation, are also the most disease-ridden people in the world.
- All nations known for their good health and exceptional vitality and longevity live on a low animal protein-high natural carbohydrate diet.

Now, before you misunderstand me on the *carbohydrate* issue, let's make it clear that I am speaking of *natural* carbohydrates. Of course, what you have heard about the harmfulness of a high carbohydrate diet is true – if you mean *refined carbohydrates* such as white sugar and white flour products. In fact, of all the underlying causes of ill health in civilized countries, I would list the refined carbohydrates, such as white sugar and white flour, and all foods made with them, as the number one cause. When I recommend a *high natural carbohydrate-low animal protein* diet I mean that the emphasis in your diet should be on fresh natural fruits and vegetables and unrefined, whole seeds and grains – all *natural* carbohydrate foods. These foods are the staples of the healthy and long-lived Hunzas, Bulgarians, Russians,

Central American Indians, etc., as you have seen in the previous chapter.

The most perfectly balanced diet is a diet rich in organically grown fruits and vegetables and raw or sprouted whole grains, seeds and nuts. Lacto-vegetarians can use raw unpasteurized milk, yogurt and homemade cottage cheese from organically raised animals. Fortified with such foods as cold-pressed vegetable oils, honey, wheat germ and bran, brewer's yeast, kelp, and dry fruits, this high *natural* carbohydrate-low animal protein diet will supply you with all the required nutrients – vitamins, minerals, trace elements, enzymes, proteins, fatty acids, carbohydrates, and other vital substances – in a natural, pure, and easily assimilated form.

6. SYSTEMATIC UNDEREATING AND PERIODIC FASTING

Would you like to learn the two most important health and longevity secrets? Here they are: 1) systematic undereating, and 2) periodic fasting (see Chapters 8 and 9 on Fasting).

Not only *what* you eat but *how much* you eat is of vital importance for your health. The latest scientific research shows that overeating is one of the main causes of man's ills, and that, conversely, *undereating* is singularly the most important health and longevity factor.

Russian statistics show that one common characteristic of all Russian centenarians is that they are all moderate eaters and have been such throughout their lives. Dr. C. M. McCay, of Cornell University, has shown that overeating is the major cause of premature aging. Systematic undereating, on the other hand, increases longevity and decreases the incidence of the degenerative diseases.

Recently, scientific studies involving earthworms, conducted by a recognized educational institution, showed that fasting worms periodically, every other day, caused them to live 50 times as long as usual!

Food eaten in excess of actual bodily need acts in the system as a poison. It interferes with digestion, causes internal sluggishness, gas, incomplete assimilation of nutrients, putrefaction, and actually poisons your whole system. Compulsive gluttons – overeaters – are usually always hungry because they are *undernourished.* "Overfed, but undernourished", as so correctly expressed by H. Curtis Wood, Jr., M. D.

Poor digestion and assimilation of nutrients caused by chronic overeating causes nutritional deficiencies. Although the compulsive glutton is fat, his body craves food because it is starving for minerals and vitamins and other needed substances. The less you eat, the less hungry you feel, because the food is more efficiently digested and better utilized. Unbelievable? But true – try it! And see the difference in the way you feel.

7. CORRECT EATING HABITS

It is important not only to select and prepare foods properly, but to eat them properly as well.

Slow eating and good mastication are essential for good health. It is far better to skip a meal than to eat it in a hurry. Good chewing increases assimilation of nutrients in the intestinal tract and makes you feel satisfied with a smaller amount of food. Saliva contains digestive enzymes; therefore, well-chewed and generously salivated food is practically half-digested before it enters the stomach.

You have been reading much about mixing foods – what foods you can and can't eat at the same meal. Whole books are written on the subject, much speculation and direct nonsense have been said, and confusion and disagreement exist. Actually, the entire food-mixing "science" can be summed up in a few lines:

1. Never eat raw fruits and raw vegetables at the same meal.
2. Eat as few different foods as possible at one meal.
3. When protein-rich foods are eaten with other foods, eat the protein foods first.

These are all the food mixing rules you need to know, rules that can be scientifically justified. Here are the scientific reasons, for these rules:

1. Raw fruits and raw vegetables require a totally different enzyme combination for their effective digestion. If you mix them in the same meal they will "confuse" your enzyme-producing glands and cause poor digestion and gas. Therefore, it would be better to make one meal of the day a *fruit meal,* where any available fresh fruit can be eaten, and another meal a *vegetable meal.* Lemon and papaya are exceptions to the rule (it seems there are always exceptions to every rule); lemon juice can be used sparingly on vegetable salads, and papaya can be eaten with any kind of food. By the way, cooked fruits after a vegetable meal seem to combine well, but why would anyone want to cook fruits?

2. There is much evidence to the effect that the fewer foods you mix at the same meal, the better will be your digestion and assimilation. Every food, every fruit or vegetable, requires a different enzyme, or enzyme combination, for the best digestion. Mono-diet – a diet system where only *one* food is eaten at a meal, a different food at each meal – would be the ideal from a health standpoint. Since few of us would ever go so far in our effort for better health as to adopt a mono-diet, a good practical rule would be: eat as few different foods as possible at any one meal.

3. Proteins need a generous amount of hydrochloric acid in your stomach in order to be properly digested. When you eat carbohydrate foods, such as vegetables and fruits, your stomach does not secrete hydrochloric acid, because it is not needed for the digestion of carbohydrates. If you first fill your stomach with predominately carbohydrate foods and then finish your meal with a protein food, the protein will remain largely undigested because of the insufficient amount of hydrochloric acid in the stomach. Therefore, it is best to always eat protein-rich foods first, on an empty stomach, when hydrochloric acid secretion will be generous; then continue with carbohydrate foods. Of course, it would be even better to eat protein foods at one meal and carbohydrate foods at another, for the reasons explained above.

By the way, we really can't talk about *protein* food or *carbohydrate* food, because there isn't such a thing. *All* natural foods contain all the food elements: carbohydrates, fats and proteins in varying amounts. You can not eat a pure protein food without some carbohydrate, or a natural carbohydrate food without some protein. White sugar, for example, is a 100% pure carbohydrate, but it is not a *natural food.* The fact that nature put proteins, fats and carbohydrates into *all* the foods intended for man's nutrition, indicates that you should not worry too much about food mixing, as long as you abide by the three simple rules, suggested above.

Finally, food should be eaten in a relaxed atmosphere and *enjoyed.* Biologically, only the foods eaten with genuine pleasure will do you any good. A peaceful, unhurried, and happy atmosphere around the table will pay good dividends in improved digestion and assimilation of food, and hence in better health.

Your health menu for a day

Here is a menu for a macrobiotic diet for optimum health and prevention of disease, based on the above principles of vitalizing nutrition:

UPON ARISING: Glass of water, plain, or with freshly squeezed lemon juice (½ lime or ¼ lemon to a glass of water).

OR: Big cup of warm herb tea. Choice of rose hips*, peppermint, camomile, or any of your favorite herb teas, sweetened with honey.

OR: Glass of freshly made fruit juice: orange, apple, pineapple, etc. No canned or frozen juices. Juice should be freshly made on your own juicer from the available fresh fruits. Juice should be diluted with water, half and half.

---

* See Chapter 16 for Recipes and Directions.

BREAKFAST:	Fresh fruits: apple, orange, banana, grapes, grapefruit, or any available berries and fruits *in season.* Cup of yogurt or homemade soured milk (made from raw, unpasteurized milk)*, preferably goat milk, with a tablespoon of sunflower or sesame meal, and/or tablespoon of flaxseed meal sprinkled over.**
OR:	Bowl of rolled oats, uncooked, with 4-6 soaked prunes (or 2-3 figs) and a handful of unsulfured raisins. Glass of unpasteurized milk or yogurt.
OR:	Handful of raw nuts (almonds, peanuts, etc.) and any fresh fruit and berries available in season.
LUNCH:	Big bowl of fresh, green vegetable salad that includes any available sprouts.* 2 or 3 middle-sized potatoes or 1 big sweet potato, boiled or baked in jackets. 1-2 slices of whole-grain bread, preferably sour-dough rye bread* with butter and mild natural cheese. Glass of yogurt or homemade soured milk.
OR:	Big bowl of fresh Fruit Salad à la Airola.*
OR:	Handful of raw nuts and fresh fruit, if not eaten at breakfast.
MIDAFTERNOON:	Glass of fresh fruit or vegetable juice.
OR:	Cup of your favorite herb tea, sweetened with honey.
DINNER:	Big bowl of fresh, green vegetable salad. (Use any and all available vegetables, including tomatoes, avacados and sprouts.)

---

* See Chapter 16 for Recipes and Directions.

** Sunflower, sesame, or flaxseed meal must be freshly made on your own seed grinder, available at department and health food stores for approximately $10.00. The best investment you will ever make!

Carrots, red beets and onions should be staples with every salad. 2-3 boiled or baked potatoes in jackets. Prepared cooked vegetable course, if desired: vegetable soup, vegetable stew, beans, peas, eggplant, artichoke, sweet potatoes, or other vegetables. Fresh cottage cheese, preferably homemade.* 1-2 slices of whole-grain bread, preferably sour rye bread. Fresh butter and slice or two of mild, natural cheese (make sure cheese is not processed or colored). Glass of yogurt or homemade soured milk.

OR: Bowl of sprouted seeds, or cereals, such as millet*, kruska*, buckwheat*, or any other whole-grain cereal (barley is especially recommended) with milk, soaked prunes, and/or unsulfured raisins. Glass of unpasteurized, fresh milk or yogurt. (This alternative only if a big bowl of vegetable salad was eaten at lunch. However, vegetable salad could be eaten twice, if desired, both for lunch and for dinner.)

BEDTIME SNACK: Glass of fresh milk, or nut-milk, or seed-milk (made in electric liquifier from seeds or nuts and water), with tablespoon of yeast and teaspoon of honey.

OR: Cup of your favorite herb tea.

OR: One apple.

---

* See Chapter 16 for Recipes and Directions.

Vital points to remember

The above menu, of course, is only a very general outline, a skeleton around which an individual diet for optimum nutrition should be built. Always keep these important points in mind:

1. The bulk of your diet should consist of fresh fruits and vegetables, preferably organically grown, most of them eaten raw. Eat as great a variety of fruits and vegetables as possible. Do not shun avacados and bananas because you may think they are fattening – they are not! If you can get papaya melon – the miracle cleansing and beautifying food – include it in your diet. A certain amount of cooked vegetables is allowed, particularly those vegetables that are not very palatable in a raw state, such as potatoes, yams, squashes, dry beans, etc. However, cooked vegetables should be used only sparingly and never *replace* the daily use of raw vegetables. At least 75% of all your food should be in a natural raw state. Fresh, leafy green vegetables and fresh fruits are packed with sun energy, with chlorophyll, enzymes, vitamins, and minerals. They are living and life-giving foods. *They contain the greatest health potential of all foods.*

2. Grains and seeds are also vitally important foods. They could be eaten raw, sprouted*, or prepared as cereals* and bread*. Millet cereal* and buckwheat cereal, kasha*, are excellent cereals. Barley, largely neglected in the U.S., is extremely nutritious grain; can be used in breads or as a cooked cereal. Eat lots of raw nuts and sunflower seeds. Sesame seeds are rich in excellent proteins and unsaturated fatty acids and could be enjoyed as homemade Halvah* or as peanut-butter-like spreads, available at health food stores.

3. Honey is a nutritional wonder of nature – use it as a substitute for sugar whenever you need a sweetener.

4. Use cold-pressed vegetable oils, such as sunflower oil, olive oil, safflower oil, linseed oil, corn oil, soy oil, wheat germ oil, etc. They are rich in vitamin F, unsaturated fatty acids, and

---

* See Chapter 16 for Recipes and Directions.

vitamin E. (Unfortunately, most American oils are over-processed. I particularly recommend to use *virgin olive oil* imported from Mediterranean countries. See Chapter 7 for danger of eating rancid oils.)

Avoid the following health destroyers:

- White sugar and white flour and everything made with them: ice cream, candies, sodas, pastries, cakes, cookies, pies, sugared desserts, etc.
- Coffee, tea, chocolate. Health food stores carry a large assortment of delicious herb teas. Carob powder is an excellent and healthful substitute for chocolate – and tastes just like it.
- Tobacco, alcohol.
- Salt, white and black pepper, mustard. When you get accustomed to eating fresh, raw fruits and vegetables you will soon find that they taste delicious even without any seasoning. If seasoning for salads or cooked dishes is desired, onions, garlic, dill, sage, watercress, paprika, red chili, and many other herb flavorings will give a wide variety of choice. Kelp, powdered or granulated, is a good salt substitute. Possibly small amounts of sea salt can be used.
- Packaged breakfast cereals. Raw oats, old fashioned or quick-cooking, may be used with milk and honey and/or raisins – children just love to eat oats this way.
- Canned, preserved, frozen and irradiated foods.

Chapter 4

Should You Take Vitamins and Food Supplements?

All nutrition experts are in complete agreement that vitamins, minerals, complete proteins, carbohydrates, essential fatty acids, enzymes and trace elements are essential both for the maintenance of good health and the prevention of disease. The disagreement and confusion starts when these experts try to determine how you should obtain all these necessary nutrients and guard yourself against nutritional deficiencies.

The official medical thinking is that a "well-balanced" diet will take care of all your nutritional needs. That is, you should get your vitamins "with a knife and fork." The usual story you hear from the average doctor is that vitamin and mineral supplements are a waste of money and absolutely unnecessary, except in cases of indicated deficiencies – and then, of course, the condition must be determined by the doctor and the vitamins prescribed by him. Our government, through the F.D.A. (Federal Food and Drug Administration), pressured by the official medicine and food processing industry, is trying very hard to put health food stores out of business by enacting a law that would make all vitamins in high potencies available only on a doctor's prescription. The F.D.A. claims that the only ones who benefit from vitamins and food supplements are the vitamin and food supplement manufacturers and retailers.

Unfortunately, there are many health writers and lecturers, particularly those who call themselves natural hygienists, who agree with this official no-vitamin-or-supplement view. They insist that taking vitamins and food supplements is unnatural, and that you can obtain all the vitamins and other nutrients you need from a well-chosen and well-balanced diet of nutritionally sound natural foods. They also claim that the addition of concentrated vitamins and supplements can be detrimental to your health.

But there is another point of view, to which an increasing number of the world's most prominent nutritionists and progressive medical researchers are turning. Their contention is that, while under ideal conditions – 100% natural, poison-free foods and a poison-free environment – you would not need any food supplements at all, under the present conditions, when the available foods are devitalized by unnatural growing methods, refining, and processing, *food supplements are imperative,* if health and vitality are to be maintained.

The poor layman is again caught between these contradictory opinions by the experts and is thoroughly confused. Should he or should he not take vitamins and food supplements? Can he get his vitamins with a knife and fork? And isn't this the most natural and sound way to acquire proper nutrition?

Changed foods and environment

Ideally, you should obtain all your nutrients in needed amounts from the foods you eat, without the addition of any food supplements. A hundred or even fifty years ago such advice would have been both sound and workable. Your grandparents ate wholesome foods which were organically grown on their own farms, without the aid of chemical fertilizers. They ate fresh fruits and vegetables from their own gardens, grown without poisonous sprays. They obtained meat, eggs and dairy products from their own healthy farm animals. They ate no processed or refined foods. The natural unrefined foods your grandparents ate contained more protein, more vitamins, and more minerals than the foods of today, grown on depleted soils and denatured and devitalized by processing and refining. The eggs they ate were fertile eggs, produced by hens that ate worms, bugs, grass, etc. Such eggs had more vitamins, more lecithin and twice as much unsaturated fatty acids as today's eggs, produced in "egg factories" by chicks that never see the sunlight – or the rooster! – and eat only chemicalized and medicated mash. The grains, the vegetables, the meat and the dairy products your grandparents ate had a higher protein content, and a higher vitamin and mineral content, and they were free from DDT, hormones, preservatives, insecticides and other chemicals and drugs, unknown 50 years ago.

Those who advocate eating regular natural foods as the only source of vitamins and other nutrients, live in a dream world of yesterday. What was yesterday's law is today's folly. It is a sad fact that due to vitamin-, protein-, and enzyme-destroying practices of the food producing and food processing industries our modern-day foods, *not only those you buy at your supermarket, but also in your health food store,* are *nutritionally inferior* to the food your grandparents ate one or two generations ago. Even those so-called organically grown foods are grown in a polluted atmosphere, are watered by polluted waters, and contain residues of toxins from fallout, etc. Also, if you buy your organic foods from your health food store, they are probably delivered there from California or Florida, are many days old, and their vitamin content thus dangerously reduced. So it really doesn't matter how well you balance your meals, or if you are a meat-eater, a vegetarian, or a raw-foodist, *you still run a risk of malnutrition if you try to get all your vitamins exclusively from the foods you eat.*

It is medically a well-known fact that even minor deficiencies of one or more of the vital nutritive factors will result in deranged chemistry in the human system, and lower the body's resistance to disease.

Thus, food supplements are necessary as a nutritional insurance against disease. Well chosen food supplements are an easy, inexpensive way to improve your diet and assure optimum health for you and your family.

The prime purpose of food supplements is to fill in the nutritional gaps produced by faulty eating habits and by nutritionally-inferior foods. Food supplements will replace in your diet the nutrients missing in food grown on depleted soils, or removed by food processing.

Protective property of vitamins and supplements

There is another good reason to supplement your diet with an extra supply of vitamins, minerals, fatty acids and other nutrients. Many of these substances have protective properties against some of today's most toxic environmental factors. They can protect you from the harmful effects of poisonous additives and residues in your food, water and air.

Vitamin C, for example, is a powerful anti-toxic agent. Huge doses of vitamin C can protect you effectively against acute poisoning from virtually any source. My friend, Dr. W. J. McCormick, of Canada, perhaps the greatest authority of the therapeutic uses of vitamin C in the world, told me that he once saved the life of a sailor who was bitten by a banana spider. Usually such a poisoning results in death within a few hours. The man was brought to his office about an hour after the sting. Dr. McCormick injected intravenously 1500 mg. of vitamin C every 10 minutes. The man left his office in three hours completely symptom-free.

Vitamin C can protect you from toxic effects of *any* bacterial or viral infection and speed recovery in *any* condition of disease. Heavy doses of vitamins C and B can modify the toxic effects of smoking and drinking. Vitamins B, D and E will help to protect you against many insecticide residues, which you just can't avoid.

Vitamins E and B_{15} will protect you against harmful effects of air pollution. As you know, the most injurious substance in polluted air is carbon monoxide. Carbon monoxide induces hypoxia by preventing oxygen from being absorbed by the lungs. Insufficient supply of oxygen to the tissues is considered to be a major cause of our worst diseases. Many scientists (O. Warburg,

H. Goldbratt, et al.) believe that a periodic lack of oxygen is responsible for the formation of cancer cells, thus being one of the causes of cancer. Vitamin B_{15}, or pangamic acid, increases the body's resistance to hypoxia, or lack of oxygen, by reducing the body's need for oxygen. And vitamin E increases cell oxygenation by as much as 60 per cent. Thus, both vitamins, E and B_{15}, can help to protect us from slow poisoning by carbon monoxide, to which we are all subjected.

One of the gravest environmental dangers to our health today is universal lead poisoning. Lead is one of the most toxic metals, and even small amounts of it can be fatal. Lead poisoning can cause damaged kidneys and liver; it can affect the nervous system, and even cause insanity. Some researchers believe that lead also can cause multiple sclerosis, interfere with fertility, and cause miscarriages and sexual impotence.[1]

Lead comes into the atmosphere mostly from automobiles which burn gasolines treated with lead. It pollutes the air, settles on soils and on the crops, and is absorbed by vegetables and fruits. In the United States, over 200 million pounds of lead enter the atmosphere from automobile exhaust pipes each year – that's one pound per capita! It has been shown that vegetables grown in gardens in a little town in New York State contained over 100 parts per million of lead – this is over 30 times the maximum permitted dose in canned foods. Even organic gardens can not escape this contamination.

It has been demonstrated that such supplements as calcium, vitamin D, vitamin C and thiamin (B_1) have a preventive and corrective effect in lead poisoning. These substances can protect you against the toxic effects of lead.

Calcium has also been shown to have a protective property against other toxic substances, for example strontium 90, to which we all are subjected in this age of atomic tests. An inexpensive food supplement, bone meal, is a good source of

---

1 See Chapter 22 in my book SEX AND NUTRITION, Published by AWARD BOOKS, New York, 1970.

easily assimilable calcium.[2]

In this polluted world of ours, where lethal poisons are lurking in all directions – the air, water, food, clothing, household items, etc. – food supplements are virtually your only available protection against the harmful effects.

Natural versus synthetic vitamins

Assuming that after reading the presentation in this chapter so far you have become convinced that supplementing your diet with vitamins and food supplements is imperative in this age of a universally toxic environment and nutritionally inferior foods, the next step would be to find out which supplements to take.

There is a great controversy in regard to the usefulness of synthetic vitamins. Most drugstore-quality vitamins are made of synthetic chemicals – they are not derivatives of natural food substances. Most vitamins sold in health food stores are concentrations of vitamins extracted from such natural sources as rose hips, green peppers and acerola (C), brewer's yeast and liver (B), fish liver oil (A and D), kelp (iodine), bone meal (minerals), etc. Most health authorities claim that synthetic vitamins are useless, ineffective and may be harmful. Most medical doctors and spokesmen for the chemical drug industry claim that "a vitamin is a vitamin is a vitamin", that synthetic vitamins have a molecular chemical structure identical to the so-called natural vitamins, and that they are just as effective in therapeutics. Who is right?

Actually, both sides are partially wrong in their mutual accusations. Some synthetic vitamins, such as ascorbic acid (vitamin C), irradiated ergosterol (vitamin D) and many synthetic B-vitamins have been successfully used in therapeutic practice,

---

2 Make sure that bone meal is imported from Southern Hemisphere, where animal bones are relatively free from strontium 90 accumulation. Health food stores carry such brands. Vitamin D, or fish liver oil, will help your body to assimilate calcium more efficiently.

particularly when large doses are required. I had long arguments with Dr. W. J. McCormick, world-famous authority on the therapeutic uses of vitamin C. I never did succeed in convincing him that natural vitamins are better than synthetic. Dr. McCormick achieved all his successful, often dramatic, healing results using only synthetic ascorbic acid in huge doses. Of course, there is much research which shows that vitamin C-complex *is* more effective than plain ascorbic acid. Bioflavonoids – rutin, citrin, and hesperidin, which always accompany vitamin C in natural foods – being *synergists,* increase the therapeutic effect of vitamin C. But this does not mean that synthetic ascorbic acid is useless. In acute conditions of poisoning or infection ascorbic acid in huge doses can be useful, preferably in combination with fresh citrus juices that contain natural bioflavonoids.

Vitamin E is another vitamin that is controversial in this respect. Proponents of natural vitamins advise taking vitamin E-rich vegetable oils, particularly wheat germ oil, because natural vitamin E occures in the form of mixed tocopherols (Alpha, Beta, Gamma, Delta). But Drs. Evan and Wilfrid E. Shute, the world's foremost authorities on vitamin E, used only isolated alpha-tocopherol in their large practice and research work. They contend that alpha-tocopherol is *the* active part of the vitamin E-complex and that the other tocopherols are not necessary.

The solution to the controversy *synthetic versus natural vitamins* seems to be that isolated and synthetic vitamins and minerals in large doses have their rightful and indispensable place in the short-term treatment of acute disease and severe deficiency conditions, but those who do not suffer from any specific disease or deficiency, but are interested in food supplements for prophylactic reasons – that is, to protect their health and to prevent disease and premature aging – should use natural vitamins and natural food supplements, such as brewer's yeast, rose hips, fish liver oils, lecithin, wheat germ, wheat germ oil, cold-pressed vegetable oils, and kelp, because in these supplements all the nutritive factors are present in their natural, balanced combinations, which is essential for better assimilation and maximum biological effect.

Dual purpose of vitamin therapy

The classic concept of vitamin therapy is that vitamins should be used only in correcting vitamin deficiencies. Doctors who are trained in this classic concept of vitamin use, prescribe specific vitamins, or vitamin-rich foods, only when a specific vitamin deficiency is indicated – and then only in the amounts necessary to build-up the recommended daily allowance, which is usually MDR, a *minimum* daily requirement.

Vitamins are catalysts, nutritive substances needed by your body in certain amounts each day for various body processes and functions. If the minimum daily requirement is not provided and vitamins are undersupplied, vitamin deficiency will result which may lead to various health disorders. When health disorders are caused by vitamin deficiencies, prescribed vitamins will correct the deficiency and cure the disorder. This is the classic concept of vitamin use.

In various research centers of the world, but particularly in Canada, USA and Russia, a totally new concept of vitamin therapy has been developed in the last few decades. Vitamins are now used in huge doses, that are *far above the actual nutritional needs.* In large doses many vitamins have a miraculous healing, stimulating and protective effect on the various body functions, an effect that is totally different from the usual vitamin activity as nutritional catalysts.

For example, you need only 100 or 200 mg. of vitamin C for the normal, healthy functions of your body. But when you take huge doses of vitamin C, we'll say 3,000 milligrams a day, it will saturate the bloodstream and all the tissues of your body and perform such miraculous things as neutralizing various toxins and poisons, killing pathogenic bacteria, speeding the healing processes, helping in the oxygenation of tissues, etc.

Another typical example is vitamin E. The official estimation of your daily requirement for this vitamin is only 10 International Units. But when taken in large doses, for example, 600 to 1,000 I.U., vitamin E assumes a drug-like role and performs a completely different activity. It increases oxygenation of the tissues by as much as 60 per cent. It dilates blood vessels and small blood capillaries and increases circulation – thus becoming a great heart saver in cases of heart condition. It has a history of dramatic effect on the reproductive organs: prevents miscarriages, increases male and female fertility, and can restore male potency.[3]

Many vitamins, such as certain vitamins from the B-complex and vitamin A, have been used in huge doses in clinical therapeutics – in doses far above the actual daily need for these vitamins. For example, the official recommended daily allowance for vitamin A is set at 5,000 USP units. But when taken in such a large dose as 100,000 units a day, vitamin A has been known to have a curative effect on many disorders, such as skin and eye diseases, infections, etc. It also has a stimulating and rejuvenating effect on many vital body processes, particularly on glandular activity, and is considered as an important life-prolongator.

What supplements to take and how much

If you are well, or relatively so, but still wish to supplement your diet for prophylactic reasons – that is, to remain healthy and prevent disease – you should not take concentrated, isolated vitamins, but should use the following foods and food supplements. These supplements will enrich your daily diet and assure you optimum nutrition. They are natural wonder foods, loaded with vital substances. Here they are:

- *Brewer's yeast* (vitamin B-complex, protein) – 2 or 3 tablespoons each day. *Note:* never use yeast intended for baking!
- *Cod liver oil,* plain, not fortified (vitamins A, F and D) – one teaspoon a day.

---

3 For scientific references on the above-mentioned properties of vitamin E see my book, SEX AND NUTRITION, Published by AWARD BOOKS, New York, 1970.

- *Raw wheat germ* (vitamin E, B-complex, protein, minerals, enzymes) – 3 to 5 tablespoons a day. *Make sure that the wheat germ is fresh, not rancid.* Fresh wheat germ tastes sweet and does not have a bitter, tangy aftertaste.
- *Rose hips,* powder or tablets (vitamin C, bioflavonoids, enzymes) – equivalent of 200 mg. vitamin C, or more, each day.
- *Wheat germ oil* (vitamin E, unsaturated fatty acids) 2 to 3 teaspoons a day.
- *Bone meal,* powder or tablets (minerals) – 2 teaspoons or 10 tables a day. (Lacto-vegetarians can use Calcium Lactate.)
- *Kelp* (iodine, minerals, trace elements) – 2 to 5 tablets a day. Use kelp granules on salads as a substitute for salt.
- *Lecithin,* granules or liquid (inositol, choline, lecithin) – 1 tablespoon a day.
- *Whey powder* (lactose, minerals, iron, B-vitamins) – 2 tablespoons a day.

For best biological value and most efficient assimilation, all food supplements should be taken with meals. Because some vitamins interfere with the absorption of others, wheat germ oil should be taken *before* meals and all other supplements *during* or *after* the meals.

Addition of these food supplements to your optimum macrobiotic diet, as outlined in Chapter 3, will not only assure you all the *known* vitamins and other nutritional factors, but also all the *unknown*, as yet undiscovered, ones. Moreover, in such natual food supplements all the nutritive factors are present in their naturally balanced combination – this is extremely important for maximum assimilation and full biological activity.

Therapeutic and protective vitamin-mineral program

The above recommendations for natural food supplements are for those who are young and relatively healthy; this is a preventive food supplement program.

Those who are *not healthy,* are over 50 years of age, and are suffering from one or more chronic conditions of ill health, lack of vitality, chronic fatigue, or signs of premature aging – and in this category would be probably found 95 per cent of all people past the half century mark – should supplement their diet with certain vitamins in higher potencies.

In addition to all the natural food supplements recommended under subtitle "What supplements to take and how much", persons who fit into the above categoryof chronically ill or half-well, should take the following additional vitamins regularly:

- *Vitamin C,* natural, with bioflavonoids – 1,500 to 2,000 mg. a day. Even more in acute conditions. Vitamin C is completely nontoxic even in huge doses.
- *Vitamin E,* alpha-tocopherol or mixed tocopherols – 600 I.U. a day. If you have not taken vitamin E before, start with 100 units a day and increase to 600 units within two weeks. If you have high blood pressure, consult your doctor before taking vitamin E.
- *Vitamin A,* natural, from fish liver oil or vegetable sources – 25,000 USP units a day.
- *Vitamin B-complex,* high potency, with B_{12}, natural from concentrated yeast – one capsule or tablet a day, or follow recommendation on the bottle.

These natural vitamins can be obtained in any health food store.

Here are four tips in regard to taking the above vitamins:

1. Divide the suggested daily amounts between three meals.

2. Take all vitamins and other supplements *with* meals, or immediately *after* meals, with the exception of vitamin E and wheat germ oil, which should be taken before meals.

3. Take all vitamins and supplements *continuously* with the exceptions of vitamins B, A and cod liver oil – these should be taken for one month, then after one month interval, taken for another month, and so on.

4. Buy three different brands of B-complex capsules at one time and take one capsule of a different brand each day. This is because every brand has a somewhat different formula, where some of the vitamins of the B-complex are in larger potencies than others. Taking a different brand every day will give you

a certain degree of assurance that whatever is undersupplied in one formula may be supplied by another formula. Read the labels for the potencies of the various B-vitamins and buy formulas where *all* different B-vitamins are well represented.

Naturally, if you are seriously ill, you should be under your doctor's supervision and you should consult him as to the advisability of taking vitamins in addition to whatever therapy he suggest. Those who take vitamin E for a heart condition should ask their doctor to establish a proper dosage for them. If your doctor is so behind the times that he does not believe in taking vitamins or in improving your health with nutritional means – for your health's sake, find another doctor. Fortunately, there is an increasing number of doctors among all healing professions who are becoming nutrition-oriented. They have to, because a rapidly increasing number of patients are becoming aware of the vital role nutrition plays in health and disease. Today's doctors have to keep abreast of patients in modern nutritional facts, or they will be losing their patients. *If doctors of today will not become the nutritionists of tomorrow, the nutritionists of today will become the doctors of tomorrow.*

Note: Recommending supplements and vitamins in large doses we do not diagnose or prescribe, but offer this nutrition information only to help you to solve your health problems in cooperation with your doctor. If you suffer from a disease and use this information without your doctor's approval, you are prescribing for yourself, and assuming the responsibility for it, which is your constitutional right to do.

Chapter 5

The Health-Building and Health-Restoring Power of Whole Grains, Seeds and Nuts

A very young health-conscious couple, barely twenty years old, with a three year old son, came to see me. I invited them for a lunch: fresh fruits, raw nuts and sesame seeds, unsulfured sun-dried figs and raisins, and yogurt – my typical meal. Both youths, and their son, took some of the fruit, but didn't touch the nuts, seeds or milk. Finally, I asked the boy if he would like to have a glass of home-made yogurt.

"No, thank you," the boy answered, very politely.

"Don't you like milk?" I asked.

"Yes, but it isn't good for me," the boy answered, very matter-of-factly.

The father looked at me with a mixed expression of apology and pride on his face for the good job of indoctrination he had done. Finally he said to me:

"Well, milk is mucus-forming – so we don't give him milk at all."

I suggested that it would be advisable for a child of this age to have some raw milk or yogurt, unless he is allergic to it. But my words fell on deaf ears. They were convinced, after reading a book on a mucus-less diet, that milk would harm their son.

Then I offered my guests some raw peanuts and almonds I was enjoying, but they refused to touch them on the grounds that "peanuts are not nuts", and, besides, "aren't all nuts acid-forming?"

Among all the great numbers of misled and confused health seekers, the most pitiful and lamentable are those who have "read *a* book". After reading one or two books on nutrition, usually by some self-styled nutrition "authority" who is just as confused as his readers, they think they know all the answers. Someone said that peanuts are not nuts, but legumes. So what? Does this revelation make them less fit as a food? Some will not touch anything grown *under the ground.* Some will eat tomatoes together with fruit because they are "acid". Some will not eat garlic or onions because they are "too strong for the mucous membranes". Some will not eat milk because "casein makes good glue". Some will not eat honey because "honey is made for the bees". Some avoid eating seeds and grains because they are "acid-forming". Some others avoid grains because they are "mucus-forming". Some hardly eat anything because they take literally the advice given by some nutrition "experts" that you should not eat proteins and carbohydrates at the same time, proteins and acids at the same time, fats and proteins at the same time, acids and starches at the same time, etc., etc. *How in the world can you avoid doing that when virtually every natural food contains ALL of the named nutrients: proteins, fats, starches, and carbohydrates?* And so on, ad infinitum.

Can you see now why I was prompted to write this *De-CONFUSION book?*

The nutritional value of whole grains and seeds

Seeds, grains and nuts are the most important and the most potent foods of all. They contain the secret of life itself, the *germ.* Through this germ in seeds the perpetuation of species is accomplished. The spark of life in the seeds is of extreme importance for man's life, his health, and his virility and reproductive capacity.

Our creator designated seeds as our most important food, because the germinating power, the life-giving energy and the magic of the seeds is the source of dynamic energy and reproductive power of man.

> "And God said, Behold, I have given you every herb bearing seed, which is upon the face of the earth, and every tree, in which is the fruit of a tree yielding seed; to you it shall be for meat."
>
> Genesis 1:29

The nutritional value of seeds and grains is fantastic. Here is just a glimpse:

- Seeds, grains and nuts are gold mines of minerals, especially calcium, phosphorus, magnesium and iron.
- They contain most of the vitamins, particularly vitamins A, B and E.
- They are nature's best source of unsaturated fatty acids and lecithin.
- They are excellent sources of proteins.

Those who minimize the importance of seeds and grains in the diet claim that grain proteins are incomplete. This is only partially true. Many seeds and nuts do contain complete proteins. Sunflower seeds, soya beans, sesame seeds, pumpkin seeds, almonds and peanuts contain complete proteins. Those grains, seeds and nuts that do not contain complete proteins can be extremely useful sources of proteins if they are eaten in combination with other protein foods, or with milk or cheese, or with vegetables. A whole-grain bread sandwich eaten with a glass of milk makes a complete protein meal, the incomplete proteins of the wheat rendered complete by the combination with the complete proteins of the milk.

Seeds and grains have been always a primary source of proteins in man's nutrition. 53 per cent of the protein consumed in the world comes from grains and seeds.

Grains and seeds – ancient foods

From the earliest primitive days of civilization, seeds have formed an important part of man's diet. Man ate seeds from fruits and wild plants, raw and untampered, even before he learned the art of cultivation. In every part of the world, by every nation and tribe, seeds and grains have always been valued as the staple foods. In Asia, the principal part of any diet has always been rice. In Scotland it has been oats. In Russia and East Europe – rye and buckwheat. In the Middle East – millet and sesame seeds. In Mexico and Central America – corn. In Europe and North America – wheat. The long-living peoples of Hunza, Bulgaria, and the Balkan countries rely heavily on grains, particularly wheat, millet and barley.

There are those who claim that man is basically a fruitarian, that fresh fruits and vegetables are man's best food. Have they ever considered why the natives living in places like Mexico, Central America, Africa or the tropical areas of the Far East, where the abundance of most delicious fruits is available year around almost free, go to great effort and hard work cultivating various grains, seeds and beans and rely on these as the dietary staple? Man has always instinctively recognized the great nutritional value of grains and seeds. The grains such as rye, wheat, oats, barley, buckwheat, millet, rice, corn, sesame seeds, peas and all kinds of beans have been the basis of human nutrition for thousands of years.

Grains – the black sheep of American nutritionists

The scare and confusion created by a few writers on the dangers of mucus-forming and acid-forming foods must be responsible for the anti-grain attitude so many American nutritionists have. Also, the American "high protein-low carbohydrate" cult has some part to play in the general disrespect that is afforded grains in America's nutritional programs. Wheat particularly has become a black sheep of American nutritionists, very unrightly so.

Europe's health authorities have a totally different view of the virtue of whole grains. The International Society for Research on Nutrition and Diseases of Civilization considers the whole grains to be the most important foods for man. I have visited and studied in many biological clinics in Europe during the past

20 years and without exception all of them use various whole grain products as the staple of their therapeutic diets.

European biological clinics specialize in therapies for a multitude of degenerative diseases. After the initial program of body detoxification by fasting and other cleansing methods, the patients are put on a special body-regeneration and health-building *optimum nutrition* program in which whole grains play an important part. Some clinics use whole soaked rolled oats in the form of müesli. Some use sprouted wheat – as, for example, in Dr. Kuhl's cancer therapy and Dr. Evers' multiple sclerosis diet. All clinics use high quality grain breads, usually sour-dough rye bread*. Nutritious cereals from buckwheat (kasha*), millet*, whole wheat (molino*); rice, or mixed cereals (kruska*) are used in all European clinics and health spas.

Professor Kollath, Dr. Bruker, Professor Dr. W. Halden and Dr. F. Grandel are some of the best-known scientists in Europe who made a special study of the value of grains in human nutrition. *They all stress over and again that whole grain products are essential for optimum health as well as for preventing and overcoming disease.*

Grains – gold mines of vitamins and minerals

Phosphorus is an important mineral for many of your body's most important functions. The utilization of calcium is closely tied to the presence of phosphorus. You also need phosphorus for the proper utilization of fat by your body. Several of the important B-vitamins can not be digested properly without a sufficient amount of phosphorus in the diet. And phosphorus is an important ingredient of the brain tissue – a mineral needed for mental power.

Fruits and vegetables are poor sources of phosphorus, although they are excellent sources of calcium. Calcium and phosphorus must be supplied by foods in about equal amounts. Those who live chiefly on fruits and vegetables and neglect eating seeds and grains, might suffer from a lack of phosphorus. Grains and seeds are nature's best source of phosphorus.

---

*See Chapter 16 for Recipes and Directions.

Iron is another vital mineral. Most American women, and an increasing number of teenagers whose staple diet seems to be processed cereals, hot dogs, doughnuts, hamburgers and cokes, suffer from iron-deficiency anemia to a great extent. Whole grains are the best source of iron; refined cereals and white bread lack organic iron, because it has been removed in the processing.

Magnesium is another mineral that is plentiful in whole grains and seeds. Magnesium is one of the most important minerals and is needed for a multitude of vital bodily functions. Seeds and grains, notably almonds, barley, lima beans, corn, wheat, oats, brown rice and Brazil and cashew nuts, are richest natural sources of magnesium.

Zinc is coming into the limelight as one of the most important trace minerals, hitherto neglected in nutrition research. Recent research from many parts of the world has linked zinc deficiency to such health disorders as infertility, prostate disorders, and retarded genital development. There are five million infertile husbands in the United States, and millions of men suffering from prostate disorders. Grains and seeds are the best natural sources of zinc. Sunflower seeds and pumpkin seeds in particular are very rich sources. Other sources are wheat bran, wheat germ, brewer's yeast and onions. Zinc, of course, is nonexistent in refined and processed grains.

Wheat has been downgraded by many health writers and even considered to be directly harmful to health. Wheat has been used in human nutrition for many centuries. The Hunza people, known as the "healthiest people in the world" use wheat as a staple in their diet. Wheat is one of the most important sources of good protein.

Although grains are excellent sources of important minerals and proteins, what puts them into a special high class as important food is their *vitamin* content. Seeds and grains are your best natural sources of two of the most important vitamins: B and E.

All nuts, legumes, seeds and unrefined grains are rich sources of most of the B-complex vitamins, especially B_1, B_2, B_6, niacin, pantothenic acid and folic acid. B-vitamins are important for the health of the nerves, for mental activity, for the digestive processes, for the heart, skin, etc. B-vitamins are also considered to be anti-aging vitamins.

Vitamin E is a truly miracle vitamin. It is called by such pet names as "reproductive vitamin", "anti-sterility vitamin", "heart-saver vitamin", "anti-abortion vitamin", and the "sex vitamin". The heart-saving property of vitamin E is due to its oxygenating ability. Vitamin E oxygenates the tissues and remarkably reduces the need for oxygen. It also dilates blood vessels and prevents excessive scar tissue formation.

Vitamin E is closely involved in many vital reproductive and sexual functions. A serious deficiency of vitamin E can cause:

- Degeneration of the epithelial or germinal cells of the testicles
- Diminished hormone production – both the sex hormones and pituitary hormones which stimulate the sex hormones
- Destruction of the sex hormones by oxidation
- Miscarriages and stillbirths
- Female and male sterility
- Premature menopausal symptoms

Vitamin E is, indeed, absolutely essential for the normal function of the reproductive system. And healthy and plentiful sex hormone production is essential for the healthy functioning of the whole body. Diminished sex hormone production is one of the main causes of premature aging.

Whole grains and seeds, and cold-pressed vegetable oils made from seeds, are the best natural sources of vitamin E. Wheat germ and wheat germ oil are particularly good sources.

Are grains and seeds acid-forming?

Yes, they are. And thank goodness for that! There are people who read one or two books on alkaline-acid balance and, not being well-versed in a difficult and confusing art of biochemistry*, become so scared of acid-forming foods that they leave out all

*I call biochemistry an art, rather than science, intentionally. Anything dealing with life and living subjects has to be more of an art than an exact science.

nuts and grains from their shopping lists. Many writers have stressed the need for more alkaline foods in the diet to balance the acid foods.

Alkaline foods are those that leave an alkaline residue in the system in the process of metabolism. Acid-forming foods are those that leave an acid residue. All fruits (even acid fruits such as oranges or lemons) and vegetables are alkaline-forming foods. Meat, fish, eggs, bread, grains and nuts are acid-forming foods; they leave an acid residue.

The problem is that we *need* acid-forming foods for optimum health just as much as we need alkaline foods. A deficiency of acid-forming foods would be just as dangerous as a deficiency of alkaline foods, if not more so. So all this fuss about acid and alkaline foods did more harm than good. Acid-forming grains, seeds and nuts are God-given foods for man – so are the alkaline fruits and vegetables. Milk and milk products are relatively neutral in this respect.

By the way, your body has what is called the "alkaline reserve" – a storehouse of alkaline substances that are used to balance the chemistry when there is too much acid present. Therefore, you don't have to worry that every meal you eat is properly acid-alkaline balanced.

To solve this alkaline-acid confusion once and for all, here is some good advice:

1. Eat the *low animal protein-high natural carbohydrate* diet recommended in this book.

2. Avoid all refined, processed, denatured, starchy and sweet foods.

3. Eat to your heart's delight of these three basic foods: 1) grains, seeds and nuts, 2) vegetables, and 3) fruits, and you'll never have to worry about acid-alkaline balance. These foods are man's most perfect foods, and they have a built-in natural acid-alkaline balance.

4. Milk, cold-pressed vegetable oils, and honey, which are all largely neutral as far as acid-alkaline rating is concerned, can complement the three basic foods.

Follow the above four rules and you will be availing yourself of a diet with the greatest potential for optimum health.

Grains, seeds and nuts – storehouses of essential fatty acids and lecithin

Unsaturated fatty acids are vitally important in the optimum diet. Lack of these fatty acids may cause eczema, dry skin, dandruff, falling hair, kidney disease, diseases of the prostate gland, and other health disorders. Grains and seeds, for all practical purposes, are the only natural sources of these unsaturated fatty acids, or vitamin F.

Cold-pressed oils that are sold in health food stores are made from various grains and seeds, such as soy beans, sunflower seeds, wheat, corn, flax seed, peanuts, sesame seeds, etc. Vegetable oils are excellent foods and should replace margarine and animal fats in your kitchen.

Lecithin is another food substance of which seeds, grains and nuts are rich sources. Lecithin is a phosphorized fat that helps in fat metabolism, is present in the body as the chief constituent of semen, brain, and nerve tissues. Endocrine glands contain large amounts of lecithin. The pineal gland is richer in lecithin than any other part of the body.

Lecithin has also another important function that has been much publicized in recent years – it is a natural emulsifier of fat and it prevents cholesterol (which is fat) from collecting in chunks and attaching to the walls of blood vessels, causing arteriosclerosis. Thus, lecithin is a good preventive of hardening of the arteries by its emulsifying effect on cholesterol.

Dr. Wilhelm Halden, of the University of Graz, Austria, reported on recent statistics which show that countries where people eat whole-grain bread and whole-grain cereals are relatively free from ischemic heart disease. Chronic oxygen deficiency in tissues is connected with coronary disease and heart attacks. Whole-grain cereals, with their rich supply of vitamins B, E, essential fatty acids and lecithin, facilitate a better utilization of oxygen and, therefore, help to prevent arteriosclerosis and heart disease. Wheat germ and wheat germ oil are the "dynamic parts" of the grains and seeds. Vitamins B and E, as well as fatty acids, are concentrated in wheat germ.

This ability of whole grains to contribute to better oxygen utilization is of particular importance to modern man. We are getting less and less oxygen into our tissues because of air pollution interfering with oxygen absorption, the lack of sufficient physical exercise, and devitalized, refined foods from which wheat germ and vitamin E have been removed.

Pacifarins and cholesterol-absorbing activity

Recent studies made by Dr. Howard Schneider, of the Institute for Biomedical Research of the American Medical Association, showed that whole wheat contains a factor which has an antibiotic effect. In animal experiments this "resistance" factor, called *pacifarins,* increased resistance to disease and prevented salmonella infections in laboratory mice.

Pacifarins are found in the outer fractions of the wheat and other grains such as corn, rye and rice – the parts of the grains that are removed from the white flour in milling process.

Also, it has been found that whole grains contain an ingredient that can actually lower cholesterol levels. Dr. Hans Fisher, of Rutgers University, reported to a recent Nutrition Conference that "wheat, barley, and oats all contain this cholesterol-absorbing activity". He stressed the fact that it is the hull portion of the whole grains that contain this cholesterol-lowering activity.

Unidentified valuable substances

In addition to all the *known* nutritive and protective substances, the whole grains, according to German scientist, Dr. Bruker, contain many *unknown,* but valuable substances that are unavailable in other foods. Research has indicated that these unidentified nutritional substances in whole grains are highly effective in preventing disease and maintaining optimum health.

Keep always in mind, however, that only the whole, fresh, unrefined grains and seeds contain all these known and unknown nutritive substances. They are largely destroyed or removed in processing and refining. You can not benefit from them by eating packaged breakfast cereals or white bread.

Best ways to use grains and seeds

All nuts should be eaten raw, never roasted. Many seeds, such as sunflower seeds, pumpkin seeds and sesame seeds should be eaten raw. Almost all seeds and grains can also be eaten in a sprouted form.*

But grains and seeds can also be eaten in the form of breads and cereals. Particularly sour-dough breads* are very beneficial and easily digested. During the natural souring process, certain substances are made more easily available for assimilation in the intestinal tract. Also, valuable lactic acids develop during the fermentation process. Lactic acid foods have been found to be excellent health foods capable of preventing diseases and even curing many illnesses, as demonstrated by Dr. Kuhl and others.

Millet, buckwheat, barley and oats make excellent cereals. Both millet and buckwheat are truly wonder foods. Millet porridge* is both a healthful and extremely delicious food. Buckwheat is rich in proteins, minerals and rutin, one of the bioflavonoids. Buckwheat porridge* is the Russian national food. Because of the rutin in buckwheat, Russians claim that buckwheat cereal will build healthy blood vessels and also help to reduce high blood pressure. There are also several ways to make uncooked cereals. See in Chapter 16 the recipe for Waerland-Kruska, an excellent, power-packed, raw cereal, full of enzymes.

SUMMARY

You can see from the above presentation that whole grains, seeds and nuts are powerful health-building and health-restoring foods. Whole grains and seeds have been the basis of human nutrition for thousands of years. There are no reasons whatsoever why they should not continue to be so. Grains, seeds and nuts are the most complete and most potent plant foods available to man. They contain proteins, carbohydrates, minerals, vitamins, essential fatty acids, enzymes, trace elements, pacifarins and other protective and nutritive substances in well-balanced proportion. Whole grains and seeds should constitute a substantial part of your macrobiotic diet for optimum health and longer life.

---

*See Chapter 16 for Recipes and Directions.

Chapter 6

Is Milk a Friend or a Fiend?

The value of milk in human nutrition has been highly disputed in the United States. Some health writers condemn milk completely, most on the grounds that:

- animal milk is intended by nature to nourish the suckling animal;
- no animal ever uses milk after the period of lactation, or after weaning;
- raw milk is dangerous because it is an excellent vehicle for pathogenic bacteria;
- today's milk is loaded with chemicals, drugs, pesticide residues, hormones, antibiotics, etc., and is unfit for human consumption.

There are others who claim that milk is an excellent and indispensible food for man, one of the most complete, protective foods. Who is right?

As often is the case, both sides are right to a certain extent, while both sides exaggerate the validity of their claims. Let's look at milk *objectively* and see if we can disperse some of the confusion.

Today's milk unfit for human consumption

Both sides agree that today's milk is unfit for human consumption. It is loaded with toxic and dangerous chemicals. Cows are treated with various antibiotics, notably penicillin and aureomycin, to combat mastitis and other diseases. Considerable residues of these drugs are found in milk. A daily dose of penicillin in milk can build up a sensitivity to the drug. If you are given a dose of penicillin later you may develop a serious reaction against it. Today's milk is also contaminated with DDT and other pesticides and herbicides, and with residues of detergents that have been used in washing milking machines and other utensils.

Pasteurization of milk was originated to protect the consumer from disease-causing bacteria that may be transmitted with milk. But pasteurization also destroys the nutritive value of the milk. It kills not only the harmful bacteria, but also all the beneficial enzymes and the beneficial bacteria present in milk. It destroys some of the vitamins. It changes the chemical structure of the protein and renders it, and the minerals, less digestible and assimilable.

Therefore, if you can not get a *high quality* milk, raw and unpasteurized, guaranteed to be from organically raised animals and 100 per cent free from chemical additives, drugs, detergents, and insecticide and herbicide residues, then you will be better off to omit milk and milk products from your diet. Only the highest quality, uncontaminated, raw milk from healthy animals can be considered as a healthful addition to your diet.

Milk – the ancient food

A review of man's recorded history reveals that man has been using animal milk for his food as far back as records go. The Aryans of Central Asia were using milk as food 4,000 years B.C. They were the first herdsmen and "milk and honey" was their prized drink – long before it was praised in the Bible. Ancient Greeks consumed goats' and mares' milk. The Bible records the use of milk throughout man's Biblical history. Milk was looked upon as an ultimate in desirability. When God promised the Land of Canaan to the children of Israel, he described it to Moses as a land flowing with milk and honey.

In various parts of the world, different animals are employed as milk suppliers, depending on climate and geographical location. Camels' milk is always popular in the Middle East and North Africa. Mares' milk is used widely in Russia and Asia. Sheeps' milk is very commonly used in Bulgaria and other Balkan countries. Goats' milk is used rather universally. But the cow has been used as man's "milk factory" more universally than any other animal.

It is noteworthy that the people we always associate with remarkable health and long life – Swedes , Bulgarians, Russians – have traditionally been heavy milk consumers. These people, particularly the long-living Bulgarians, use very little meat, but consume large quantities of milk and milk products.

European nutrition research and milk

Virtually all European nutritionists and medical researchers, who have done research on the value of milk in human nutrition, recommend milk as a principle part of the diet.

One of the most famous European health-systems is the Waerland Health system. It is very popular in many European countries and many natural healing clinics in Europe use the Waerland diet program in the treatment of a multiplicity of diseases. Milk is an important part of the Waerland diet.

Dr. Werner Zabel is one of the most famous European nutrition-oriented doctors. He is a cancer specialist and director of his own famous clinic in Berchtesgaden. In his clinic all patients are given what Dr. Zabel calls an *optimum diet.* Number one source of protein in this diet is what Europeans call "kvark", a homemade cottage cheese, made from low-fat, raw milk. Kvark is made in the following manner. Lactobacillus acidophilus culture is added to fresh raw milk. When the milk is coagulated by the action of the bacteria, the cream that settles on the top is removed and all the curds are separated from the milk by running it through a fine sieve. The resulting low-fat cottage cheese is a very natural, unheated product, a very easily digested protein of the highest biological value. A pint of such cottage cheese contains about 100 grams of protein.

Of course, in European clinics, they also use the whey, which is the liquid that is left over after the curds are taken away. Whey is an extremely important food. It contains the minerals of the milk and the milk sugar, lactose. It also contains a very important substance, *orotic acid,* known to help in the regeneration of a damaged liver.

The latest European medical opinion is that milk, and particularly soured acidophilus milk, is a most effective food in regenerating the human intestinal tract and correcting digestive disorders and constipation.

The importance of milk in human nutrition is stressed by the International Society for Research on Nutrition and Diseases of Civilization, of which I spoke before. This foremost authority on nutrition in the world today considers high quality milk and homemade cottage cheese as an essential part of the optimum diet for people in our hemisphere.

Is yogurt a "wonder-health" food?

Indeed it is. Yogurt is a true wonder food, if there ever has been such a thing. Among its many wonderful properties, here are a few most important ones:

- It contains high quality proteins, minerals, vitamins and enzymes. It contains all the known vitamins, including the hard-to-get ones, D and B_{12}.
- It is a pre-digested food changed to this state by the action of special bacteria that it contains, lactobacillus bulgaris. Because of this, yogurt is digested and utilized in the body twice as fast as ordinary milk.
- It prevents putrefaction in the large intestine, a cause of disease and premature aging. Lactobacillus bulgaris destroys

putrefactive bacteria and cultivates the growth of "friendly" acidophilus bacteria that help in manufacturing vitamins B and K in the intestines and also assist in the assimilation of nutrients from the foods.

- It effectively prevents constipation.
- Yogurt is a natural *antibiotic.* It has been reported that an 8-oz. jar of yogurt, refrigerated for a week, provides an antibiotic value equal to 14 units of penicillin. Yogurt kills such virulent bacteria as *amoeba, typhus, S. dysenteriae, E. coli, streptococcus, staphylococcus,* etc.

And the wonder of yogurt is that while it destroys the dangerous, pathogenic bacteria, it is not harming the beneficial bacteria. Quite to the contrary – it assists in their growth!

The latest news on yogurt from Europe is that the use of special cultures of *Lactobacillus bifidus, Lactobacillus acidophilus,* and other human *symbionts* in preparing of yogurt improves the therapeutic value of yogurt and makes it more effective in restoring and keeping the intestinal tract in a healthy condition.

Of course, also the other forms of cultured milks, such as ordinary soured milk, acidophilus milk, or kefir, possess similar health-promoting and disease-preventing properties.

Colonic hygiene – the secret of perpetual health and eternal youth

Of all the "secrets" which man has tried to find in his endless search of means and ways of improving his health and prolonging his life, none is more scientifically established than one which is based on the premise that the *colonic hygiene* – or the clean and efficiently functioning digestive, assimilative and eliminative system – is the real secret of perpetual health and eternal youth.

Ilja Metchnikoff, the eminent Russian bacteriologist, made a revolutionary discovery at the turn of the century. He proved by experiments as well as by statistics that auto-toxemia (self-poisoning) through putrefaction of metabolic wastes in the large intestine is the main cause of premature aging as well as a direct or contributing cause of the development of many diseases.

Your intestines house billions of bacteria which help your digestive system to break down the food you eat and assist in the digestion and assimilation of nutrients. Some of these bacteria are called "the friendly bacteria", like the *acidophilus or bifidus;* some are called "the unfriendly bacteria", which are *putrefactive* bacteria. For optimum health it is imperative to maintain a good balance between these bacteria. When your diet is unbalanced, as in the case of too much animal protein and over-refined, constipating foods, the balance in the intestinal flora will be distorted. Harmful, unfriendly bacteria will take over and the result will be sluggish bowels and constipation. The toxins, or poisons, created by bacterial metabolism and putrefaction, remain in the intestines and, as a result of prolonged constipation, are absorbed by the blood stream and consequently poison the whole organism.

Metchnikoff claimed that sour-milk or yogurt-eating peoples of Bulgaria, Russia and East European and Balkan countries live longer and enjoy better health throughout their long lives because *their intestinal tract is clean and healthy.* Yogurt supplies lactic acid which kills the putrefactive bacteria. It also supplies the lactose which is a natural food of the beneficial acidophilus bacteria, thus helping their growth.

Whey – Swedish answer to yogurt

Whey possesses qualities very similar to yogurt in a somewhat more concentrated form. It is the yellowish liquid left after cottage cheese is made. It has been scientifically established that using whey regularly will prevent internal sluggishness, gas, bowel putrefaction and constipation. Whey has a similar effect on the digestive tract to that of yogurt. It particularly helps in retention of minerals in the system, especially calcium. In addition to being an excellent internal cleanser, whey is an excellent food.

In Sweden, whey is never thrown away; in fact, it is a national food. It is dehydrated and made into whey cheese (mess-ost) and whey butter (mess-smör). Whey cheese and whey butter are sold in every Swedish food store. Swedes eat these foods daily – you can find them on every Swedish table. In the United States you can buy imported whey cheese in some better delicatessen stores. In one health food store in Santa Monica, California, I found whey cheese made by American Swedes in the state of Washington. Health food stores also sell whey powder or whey tablets.

Here are a few nutritional data on Swedish whey cheese (I presume American whey powder has a similar content):

- 77% of it is pure *lactose* – the active factor responsible for its favorable influence on the intestinal tract.
- It has only 3.6% of butterfat as compared with 25 to 40% for ordinary cheese.
- It has 6 times more iron than beef, twice as much as beans or eggs and 50% more than liver.
- It has 10 times more vitamin B_1 than ordinary cheese, twice as much as beef, and 5 times as much as milk. Whey contains almost as much B_1 as the richest natural source of the B-vitamins – brewer's yeast. Yeast – 16 mg. per 100 gm.; whey – 15.5 mg.
- It has 7 times as much vitamin B_2 as beef, 10 times as much as milk, and 20 times as much as whole wheat flour.

And, whey cheese is one of the most delicious foods, too! Don't you think it would be wise to incorporate this miracle milk product – whey – into your daily diet?

Lactose – natural food for intestinal flora

Dr. Boris Sokoloff has made extensive research on the intestinal flora, and his conclusion is that the secret of remaining healthy is to provide the beneficial bacteria in the intestines with the proper food. "Drink plenty of acidophilus milk", is Dr. Sokoloff's advice. Lactose is the natural food for the beneficial acidophilus bacteria. And note this: *lactose appears only in milk* There is no other way to obtain this form of sugar. Lactose is not digested in the stomach or small intestines, but is transported undigested into the large intestine where it is used as food for the beneficial acidophilus bacteria. In addition to helping establish healthful intestinal balance, lactose aids the body in another way: it assists in the assimilation of several important minerals – chiefly calcium, phosphorus and magnesium. Experiments have demonstrated that giving lactose along with bone meal has doubled the calcium retention from the bone meal.

Milk versus meat as a protein source

I am often asked: "You are against animal proteins, yet you recommend milk. Isn't milk an animal protein?"

First, I am not against animal proteins – I am against *too much* animal protein. Chapter two of this book makes it clear that the optimum diet with the greatest potential for good health, prevention of disease and long life is a *low animal protein-high natural carbohydrate diet.* This is the diet all people known for their good health and long life traditionally exist on.

Of all animal proteins, milk is biologically much preferable to others. *First,* milk protein, casein, is the highest grade animal protein known to man. Milk protein is more "complete" than other kinds of animal protein – i.e. it has the highest biological value, because it has the best combination of essential amino acids and the right amounts of each amino acid in proportion to the others. Because of this, milk protein is very easily digested and more fully utilized than any other form of animal protein, including eggs and meat.

The *second* advantage of milk, as compared to meat, is that it does not add purines and uric acid to the body. Meat protein is a burden to the body because it contains toxic waste materials and also leaves a toxic residue in the body during the digestive process.

Is milk mucus-forming

The mucus-scare again! Yes, milk is mucus-forming. But the harm of mucus-forming foods is over-emphasized and exaggerated. Except in cases of allergy or extreme sensitivity to milk, a healthy body will take care of any extra mucus that the milk may possibly produce.

Besides, you need mucus! Mucus is an extremely beneficial and absolutely necessary substance to keep your stomach and bowel linings and all the internal membranes in good health. Your body is equipped with special glands that produce mucus to lubricate all the internal organs and membranes. Mucus is particularly needed for protecting the lining of the stomach from the corrosive effect of the strong acids secreted by the digestive glands. Mucus is also needed in great quantities during all acute conditions of infection, such as colds, for example. Mucus protects all your internal membranes and tissues from bacterial attack. Mucus also speeds the healing process in every condition where the internal membranes and linings are damaged.

It is conceivable that nature provided special foods for man that stimulate mucus production and thus keep all the internal linings well lubricated. Grains and nuts are mucus-producing foods. And so is milk. And so are the vitamins A, C and E. Thank goodness for this! We would not live long without mucus-producing foods; we would shrivel and dry out.

This is not to say that some people may not be extra sensitive to mucus-producing foods. They should, of course, exercise caution. *Moderation* is good advice in every phase of nutrition, including the mucus-producing foods, of which cows' milk is one. Used in moderation, however, milk can be enjoyed without any fear as far as mucus is concerned by an average person who is not suffering from milk allergy.

Is goats' milk better than cows' milk?

Goats' milk is better than cows' milk as a human, and especially as an infant food, because its protein and mineral ratio is more similar to human mothers' milk. Goats' milk has more niacin and thiamine, and better quality proteins than cows' milk. Also, the fat in goats' milk is naturally homogenized, and is therefore more easily digested and assimilated. Incidentally, goats' milk is *not* mucus-forming.

Thomas Parr, the Englishman who reportedly lived to be 152 years old, was examined after his death by the attending physicians. The autopsy revealed that his internal organs, and particularly his digestive tract, were in an extraordinarily healthy condition, just like those of a man 100 years younger. Mr. Parr's diet virtually throughout his life consisted almost entirely of goats' milk, goats' milk cheese, whey and raw vegetables.

SUMMARY

After reviewing all the beneficial properties of milk, particularly in the form of yogurt, whey and other soured milks, it would appear that nature may very well have intended that man should use these foods for his nutritional needs. And why not, knowing, for example, how extremely beneficial lactose is for the health of your digestive, assimilative and eliminative tract, and that milk is the *only* food which contains lactose!

Be it as it may, *milk has been used as a basis of diet by billions of people throughout man's history.* Newest research confirms the health-building and disease-preventing properties of milk, and particularly yogurt and acidophilus milk. It may be wise to include milk, yogurt, whey and homemade cottage cheese as an essential part of your optimum diet for optimum health.

But remember: only the highest quality milk can be considered as suitable for human food. It must come from healthy animals, raised on organic farms which use no chemical fertilizers; it must be raw, unpasteurized; and it must be 100 percent free from chemical additives and residues of drugs, hormones, antibiotics, detergents and pesticides.

Chapter 7

The Health Hazard of Rancid Foods

We all object to industrialized, processed and refined foods because of the lowered nutritional value. We tend to regard food processors as diabolic monsters who deliberately remove health-giving nutrients from the natural foods and sell us devitalized, inferior products. We forget that the original purpose of some of these basic refining and processing methods was actually an attempt to protect foods from rapid deterioration and improve their storage property. Fresh, unprocessed foods are *extremely perishable.* For example, leafy vegetables lose 50 per cent of their vitamin C *in just one day* after they have been harvested! Whole wheat flour turns rancid in *just a few days.* So let's not judge food processors too hard. While their main reason for processing and denaturing foods is to prolong their shelf life, there is a certain degree of attempt to protect the consumer from deteriorated, rancid and spoiled foods.

Health hazard of unprocessed foods

Those of us who are convinced of the danger of eating processed and refined foods, and eat only whole, unprocessed, so-

called health foods, often forget that natural, unprocessed foods, especially fats and oils, are extremely perishable.
Here are a few examples:

- Raw wheat germ is fresh, wholesome and edible only about 4 days – maximum a week – after it is made.
- Even storing wheat germ at low temperatures does not prevent it from oxidation and rancidity, but only slows it down.
- Most vegetable oils turn rancid in a matter of weeks, especially if they are kept in transparent glass containers at room temperature.
- Flaxseed oil is known to become rancid just a *few hours* after it is pressed.
- Butter and margarine keep fresh only two months.
- Most seeds and nuts with a high oil content turn rancid in less than a year. Hulled sesame seeds, which contain over 50% fat, keep fresh less than 6 months.
- Flaxseed meal, sunflower seed meal, or sesame seed meal keep fresh only a few days. After one week they are rancid to the point of being harmful.

Danger of processed, commercial fats

The above list is in reference to so-called natural health foods that can be hazardous to health, if not fresh. Fats and oils are, however used extensively in production and processing of regular, supermarket-type foods. Doughnuts, roasted nuts and seeds, bakery foods, pies, potato chips, deep-fried restaurant foods, commercially fried chicken – all these and many other typical American foods are made with, or fried in, rancid fats and oils. Often the same oil is used over and over, heated and reheated, as, for example, in cooking doughnuts or nuts. The roasted peanuts you eat are actually not roasted; they are cooked in oil which has been heated to an extremely high temperature.

Practically all commercial food fats and oils are made from rancid sources that should not be considered fit for food. Rancid oils are usually reclaimed for use by refining, deodorizing and bleaching, but, although the rancid smell and taste can thus be removed, the harmful chemical substances, created during oxidation, still remain in such oils.

Rancidity is the chemical change in the fat or oil produced by the combination of oxygen from the air with the unsaturated fatty acids in the oil. During such oxidation, a variety of chemical substances is formed. Oxygen is readily absorbed by the oil, where it breaks a double bond to unite with the fatty acids in the oil to form what are called peroxides. The importance of the double bonds is that they give certain fatty acids the properties known as vitamin F activity. The peroxides that are formed break down, especially in the presence of moisture, into substances called aldehydes, which give the rancid oils their characteristic odor and flavor.

The rancidity process in oils starts immediately after the oil is made. First there is an induction period during which the oils slowly but steadily take up oxygen to form the peroxides. The oxidation process speeds up as the aldehydes are formed. After the initial induction period, *rancidity can not be prevented,* even if the supply of oxygen is cut off. This fact is of great importance, because many people take certain vegetable oils in a capsule form thinking that oil in capsules is safe from oxidation, and consequently from rancidity. If the oil had been exposed to the air prior to capsuling – during the so-called induction period – then the peroxides that had already formed in the oil will continue to break down into the products responsible for rancidity, *even when oil is packaged in a capsule form.*

To prevent rancidity in oils, processors treat the oils with various chemicals to remove the most easily oxidized materials. Steam and vacuum processes are used, in addition to filtering and adding antioxidants of various kinds. Citric acid, tartaric acid, phosphoric acid, and ascorbic acid have been used as antioxidants.

Natural antioxidants

Natural seeds, grains and nuts are well protected by shells, hulls or coverings against air and light reaching the oil. Whole seeds can be stored for extended periods of time without any sign of rancidity unless the seeds have become bruised or broken. In addition, seeds contain natural antioxidants which protect the oils from oxidation and rancidity. Vitamin E, carotines and phospholipids, which are contained in varying amounts in all oil-bearing foods, act as antioxidants. Sesame oil contains an unidentified substance which gives it unusual stability. Unfortunately, most of these natural antioxidants are destroyed in commercial processing and refining of oils.

Vitamin E is considered to be a particularly effective natural antioxidant. The vegetable oils with the highest content of vitamin E are afforded the best protection from rancidity.

The vegetable oil that turns rancid faster than any other oil is flaxseed oil. It is known to become rancid just a few hours after it is made. It contains very little vitamin E – less than any other vegetable oil.

The following true story illustrates vividly how common people, guided by instinct and taste, protect themselves from harmful foods.

The place: a small town in East Germany. The period: a few decades back. The time: 6 o'clock in the morning. House wives are awakened in the early morning by the musical street vendor slowly moving through every street in his horse-drawn buggy. He stops at every block. Housewives rush to him with their small containers and buy just a few ounces, *a day's supply,* of flaxseed oil. A fresh supply of flaxseed oil is pressed each night and sold every morning. Experience has taught the housewives that oil over a day old is not suitable for eating. By the way, flaxseed oil is the most commonly used food oil in Eastern Europe.

Why rancid foods are harmful

A German scientist, Dr. H. Anemueller, is a foremost authority on the subject of rancidity and perishability of natural foods. He has written several books on the subject. Here's what he says about rancid foods:

"During the oxidation process harmful chemical substances are produced in foods. These substances irritate the delicate linings of the stomach and intestines. Prolonged use of rancid oils or foods can under some conditions have a carcinogenic effect – in other words, they may cause cancer by the virtue of being strong chemical irritants."

Scientists agree that besides altering the odor and the flavor in oils and foods, the products of the oxidation which cause rancidity are detrimental to health. Here is a partial list of what rancid oils and foods can do:

- The digestion of oils by pancreatic enzymes is clearly retarded by rancidity. The body can not effectively digest or assimilate rancid oils.
- Animal studies show that the products of oxidation in flax-seed oils are found to be lethal to rats.
- Oxidation destroys vitamins E, F, A and carotene in the oil.
- Eating rancid oils or rancid foods causes destruction of vitamins E, A and F stored in the body, or supplied with other foods, thus causing nutritional deficiencies.
- Rancid oils can irritate stomach and bowel linings and cause acute and chronic disorders.
- Rancid oils can cause cancer. Drs. Rowntree and Barrett, of the University of Pennsylvania, demonstrated the carcinogenic effect of cereal oils in their rancid state. Every rat fed a sample of rancid wheat germ oil developed malignant tumors.

Rancid health foods are anything but "healthy"

Wheat germ, wheat germ oil, cold-pressed vegetable oils, sunflower seeds, flaxseed meal, sesame seeds, raw nuts, whole grain flour and bread – these are the popular health foods millions of health-conscious people gorge upon in good faith that these wonder foods will assure their good health and prevent diseases. These foods have been recommended and popularized by many health writers and lecturers. They are sold in every health food store. Can these foods be considered health foods?

Since you have acquired this book, and used some hard-earned dollars to do so, in the hope of finding some useful, beneficial information on today's confusing and controversial issues of nutrition and health, I have to tell you the facts as they are. And the facts are that you will be far better off if you leave alone some of these popular foods – not because there is anything wrong with these foods per se, but because of the way these products are produced and marketed in the United States. *You just can not obtain them fresh enough to be considered suitable for human consumption.* In fact, some of the wheat germ, wheat germ oil or sunflower seeds I have bought in health food stores I wouldn't give to my own dog!

Wheat germ

Fresh raw wheat germ tastes delicious and very *sweet.* It has no bitter, unpalatable acrid taste. The best way to find out if wheat germ is fresh or rancid is to take a mouthful and chew for a half minute or so, then swallow. If it leaves a harsh, bitter taste in the mouth and a burning sensation in the throat – *it is rancid!*

I have met many people during my seminars who have been eating wheat germ for as long as 20 years and always thought this bitter aftertaste is a natural, inherent characteristic of wheat germ. They have never tasted fresh wheat germ!

Wheat germ keeps fresh a *maximum* of one week after it is made. Even after three days it already begins to taste rancid. There is no way you can avoid the process of oxidation if wheat germ has been exposed to air for as little as a few hours. I have never succeeded in buying vacuum packed raw wheat germ which has not been rancid, probably because it was already rancid before it was vacuum packed. Every time I ask health food store attendants if the wheat germ is fresh I hear the same comment, "Yes, we just received it from the distributor a few days ago." They have no way of knowing how long it has been stored by the wholesale distributor, or when it was actually made by the producer. So now I never buy wheat germ unless I taste it first. And since I do taste it first, *I have not been eating any wheat germ, to mention, for the past 6 years.* And how I miss it! In Canada I used to buy wheat germ from a health food store which purchased it directly from a nearby mill three times a week – so I know how fresh wheat germ should taste.

If you can't buy fresh wheat germ, you will be safer without it. How I hate to give you this advice, knowing that fresh wheat germ is a real wonder health food, loaded with excellent proteins, vitamins B and E, minerals and enzymes!

Wheat germ oil

Wheat germ oil is another popular health food. If it could be obtained fresh it would be a miracle health food. It is the richest source of vitamin E and excellent unsaturated fatty acids. It possibly contains, in addition to vitamin E, an unidentified substance that has a beneficial, rejuvenative and restorative effect on endocrine glands and on the reproductive organs, as some research indicates.

It is almost impossible, however, to obtain wheat germ oil which isn't rancid. I have thrown bottle after bottle of expensive wheat germ oil into the garbage can after bringing it from the store and then discovering that it was rancid. Sometimes, the oil tastes fresh, but starts to acquire a rancid taste after a few days of use, even when stored in the refrigerator.

Remember, not only are all the beneficial vitamins, including the all-important vitamin E, destroyed when wheat germ oil turns rancid, but the harmful chemicals created in the oil by the process of oxidation can cause many serious health disorders, including cancer.

Cold-pressed vegetable oils

Read the labels! I am sure there are not quite as many crooks in the health food producing business as in regular food processing business, but there are some. You have to be an avid label reader, even in health food stores, if you don't want to be "taken". Have you seen labels stating *cold-processed* oil? This is not the same as *cold-pressed,* although many an unsuspecting buyer may think so. Cold-pressed means that the oil was actually pressed out from the seeds by pressure without heat. *Cold-processed* may mean that the oil is obtained by chemical solvent extraction. Oil-bearing seeds are dumped into a mineral oil solvent which draws out the vegetable oil from the seeds. The oils are then separated by another chemical process. Small amounts of the chemical solvent are carried over to the finished product. These chemical residues can be harmful. Wheat germ oil is often made by this *cold-processed* method. This kind of oil was used in experiments where rats fed wheat germ oil developed malignant tumors in the intestines.

Another danger with vegetable oils in the United States is that they are usually sold in transparent glass bottles. Light speeds the processes of deterioration in the oil and accelerates the development of rancidity. In European health food stores all vegetable oils are sold in metal containers. Containers should not be galvanized, because oil dissolves zinc from the galvanizing, which also accelerates the development of rancidity. Heat does the same. Why are the vegetable oils sold in health food stores not stored in the dark of the refrigerator?

Sunflower seeds

Here is a miracle food that could make a terrific contribution to health if only it were available fresh. Hulled sunflower seeds deteriorate rapidly. Also, during the hulling process many seeds are broken or bruised. These damaged seeds deteriorate even faster. Next time you buy a package of sunflower seeds, look closely at the seeds and see how many are yellow, brown, dark or otherwise different from the normal light-gray color? Separate the damaged seeds – sometimes as much as 25 per cent of all the seeds may be damaged! – and try to eat them. Then you will know how rancid sunflower seeds taste!

I was raised on sunflower seeds in Europe, and appreciate their tremendous nutritional value. In spite of this, I have not eaten sunflower seeds for years, because I could not find anywhere in the United States sunflower seeds fresh enough to be edible.

Sesame seeds

When I lived in Toronto, Canada, I used to buy sesame seeds at a Chinese Market – this was before there were any health food stores. Once I went to buy my seeds (it was in May), but the Chinese attendant shook his head with a smile: "We only sell sesame seeds between September and April. Sesame seeds keep fresh only 6 or 7 months after they have been harvested. Come back in the fall, when the new crop comes in."

Sesame seeds contain over 50 per cent oil and, therefore, are extremely perishable. You can judge their freshness by the color: fresh sesame seeds are light yellow, while old and rancid seeds acquire a muddy gray look. Also, rancid sesame seeds taste bitter. Before you buy sesame seeds, taste them. If they taste bitter, do not buy.

Sunflower seed meal, flaxseed meal, sesame seed meal

Health food stores carry these foods, but I have yet to find one package which is edible. These seeds are extremely rich in oils, and as soon as they are ground, the oxidation process sets in. In a few days these foods are rancid enough to be considered harmful.

Raw nuts

Most nuts keep fresh *in shells* for as long as a year. Shelled nuts deteriorate gradually, some more rapidly than others. Almonds are usually quite safe. Walnuts and cashews are less durable. Especially bad are nuts which are not whole, but sold as pieces, the so-called diced nuts.

The really safe way to eat nuts is to buy them in shells and do your own cracking.

What can you do?

To sum up, there is grave danger in eating rancid foods and rancid oils. Natural, unprocessed foods are extremely perishable. Rancid foods have lost most of their nutritive value. In addition, the chemical substances which are produced during the oxidation process can irritate delicate linings of the stomach and intestines and have a carcinogenic effect – that is, they may cause cancer. They may also cause many other acute and chronic disorders.

Here are seven rules that will help to protect you from the danger of eating rancid foods:

1. Buy and eat only *really fresh* products.
2. *Taste them!* Rancid foods have a changed taste.
3. Do not buy milled products of oil-rich seed. Buy a little seed grinder (for about $10.00) and grind your own seeds.
4. Buy nuts *in shells* and crack them just before eating.
5. Never use potato chips, doughnuts, regular peanut butter, or other foods which are made with rancid oils.
6. Keep oils and all oil-rich seeds, nuts and other foods in the *refrigerator.* Darkness and cool temperature slows down the oxidation (although it does not prevent it).
7. If you can not get fresh, non-rancid wheat germ, wheat germ oil, vegetable oils, sunflower seeds, or other seeds and nuts – *do not use them.* You will be far better off without them.

Advice to health food stores

Rancid health foods is a very serious matter. I know a score of health food store owners and in my experience most of them are wonderful dedicated people, motivated by the sincere desire to make an honest contribution to the better health of our people. I am sure that if they realized the seriousness of the rancidity problem, they would do all in their power to remedy it. But only aroused public demand can effectively force the food producers and processors to supply real *health* foods, free from rancidity. If the public stops buying rancid wheat germ or other rancid foods, the producers will soon develop better and faster delivery methods to assure freshness. After all, papayas keep edible only a few days, but we are able to get them fresh, delivered daily by jets from Hawaii. This can be done with wheat germ and wheat germ oil if strong enough demand is created and voiced.

Here are seven points of friendly advice to health food store operators, which can help them to better serve their customers and protect them from rancid foods.

1. Be first in your area – buy and install in your store an effective, adjustable electric mill that will perhaps cost $150-200. Buy whole seeds and grains *in bulk* and *grind fresh meals and flours while the customer is waiting.* The price of the mill will be returned manifold in just a few months. For example, you pay $8.00 for 100 lb. of hard wheat and sell if for $30.00 ground into whole wheat flour. Not to mention the "fringe" benefits in terms of better health for your grateful customers. Such a mill can be used to grind fresh sunflower meal, flaxseed meal, sesame meal, all grains, etc.

2. Do not accept wheat germ or wheat germ oil from the wholesale distributors unless it is *dated* as to the date of production. See that it is fresh.

3. Demand that vegetable oils are packaged in metal container or in dark glass bottles.

4. Store all seeds, wheat germ, vegetable oils, nuts and grains in the refrigerator at all times.

5. If you notice that too large a percentage of sunflower seeds in a package is rancid (yellow, brown or dark colored seeds), return the shipment back to the wholesale distributor or producer.

6. If there is in your vicinity a large commercial flour mill, you may make special arrangements for direct delivery of freshly made wheat germ to your store twice a week.

7. Let your customers taste oil-containing food before they buy it. If it is rancid, I am sure you don't want to sell it to them – return it to the distributor. Isn't it better to keep a happy and healthy customer than to sell him an inferior product?

Chapter 8

Facts, Fads and Fallacies About Fasting

Fasting is the oldest therapeutic method known to man. Even before the advent of the "medicine man" and the healing arts, man instinctively stopped eating when feeling ill and abstained from food until his health was restored. Or perhaps he learned this, the most efficient means of correcting any disease, from animals, which always fast when not feeling well. Certainly, nature provided man with a definite protective and health-restoring alarm signal, which suggests to him to abstain from eating by taking away his appetite for food.

Throughout the long medical history fasting has been regarded as one of the most dependable curative and rejuvenative measures, Hippocrates, "the Father of Medicine", prescribed it. So did Galen, Paracelsus, and all the other great physicians of old. Paracelsus called fasting "the greatest remedy; the physician within". Fasting was practiced by many great thinkers and philosophers, such as Plato and Socrates, to "attain mental and physical efficiency". Most Eastern philosophers and super-yogis, known for their long life, mental efficiency and spiritual awareness, fast regularly, along with their meditation, to attain long life and a high level of spirituality.

With the advent of modern, drug-oriented medicine, fasting has fallen into disregard in the eyes of the orthodox practitioners. We are living in the age of "diets", when almost half of the population is constantly trying to "reduce" by way of countless restricted diets of every imaginable description. But the classic, and the best form of reducing – the total abstinence from food, or fasting – is seldom tried. Those who employ fasting, either for healing or reducing, are still looked upon as crackpots, quacks, and health-nuts, to say the least.

Medical science rediscovers fasting

Happily all this has been rapidly changing. Doctors have stopped laughing and started investigating. Many scientific studies and clinical tests are being made, particularly in Europe, to determine the prophylactic, therapeutic, and rejuvenating properties of fasting. The Karolinska Institute in Stockholm, the world-famous medical research institution, has made clinical studies and experiments with fasting under the direction of Drs. P. Reizenstein and J. Kellberg. They employed fasts up to 55 days in their studies.

Perhaps these studies were inspired by the famous Swedish fast marches of 1954 and 1964 which are described in detail in my book *HEALTH SECRETS FROM EUROPE* (published by Parker Publishing Co., Inc., West Nyack, N.Y. 1970). In these experimental fast marches, which made headlines in the world press, first 11 and then 19 men walked from Gothenburg to Stockholm, a distance of over 325 miles, in 10 days. Throughout each march the participants fasted – didn't eat any food at all! Dr. Lennart Edrén, D.D.S., who directed the fast marches, said after the 1954 fast march:

"This fast was the first in the series of experiments to determine the effects of total fasting under severe conditions of stress. If we find out that fasting will not cause any damage to the body, but will, on the other hand, exert a beneficial, revitalizing, cleansing and rejuvenating effect on bodily functions, it will supply invaluable information for healthy as well as for sick people. The healthy will be encouraged to fast in order to rejuvenate and increase vitality, and the sick to cure their ills. This experiment proved to the world the preventive and the therapeutic potentials of fasting."

Dr. Karl-Otto Aly, M.D., one of the leading biologically-oriented doctors in Sweden, and one of the participants of the fast marches, said:

"The march clearly showed that man can live for an extended period of time without food, even accomplish a hard physical effort while fasting. The general expressed feeling among participants was that they felt stronger and had more vigor and vitality after the fast than before it . . . .The prime goal of these experiments was to stimulate scientific institutions to engage in a thorough and objective scientific study of fasting and its prophylactic and therapeutic potentials, so that fasting will be generally incorporated into the growing arsenal of medical practices for the benefit and blessing of a disease-ridden mankind."

Dr. Ragnar Berg, one of the greatest nutrition experts in the world and Nobel Prize winner, said after the Swedish fasts of 1954 that the successful completion of this unprecedented fast was no suprise to him. He had fasted himself many times and also had supervised many fasts, including one of over one hundred days. He called the Swedish fast marches a "great scientific success".

Are Waerland is another great Swedish health pioneer who practiced and advocated fasting. Fasting is a standard initial cleansing method in the world-famous Waerland Healing System. (Incidentally, I have been extremely fortunate to have had both Dr. Ragnar Berg and Are Waerland as my teachers and close friends.)

In Germany, there are hundreds of clinics, operated by medical doctors, where fasting is now employed on a grand scale. For example, at the Buchinger Sanatorium in Bad Pyrmont fasting is used initially in almost every condition of ill health. Well over 80,000 fasts were supervised by Dr. Otto H. F. Buchinger and his father, both medical doctors, during their 50 years of practice.

Another great fasting specialist in Germany is Dr. Werner Zabel.

"Together with fever and optimal nutrition, *fasting is man's oldest and best healing method"*, said Professor Zabel.

249 days on a liquid fast!

At the Stobhill General Hospital in Glasgow, Scotland, fasting was clinically tested with remarkable results. One 54-year-old woman with a painful arthritic condition and grossly overweight, was put on a liquid fast for 249 days and lost 74 of her 262 pounds. Her arthritis cleared up completely, too!

The rejuvenating effects of fasting

The therapeutic effect of fasting is very well documented by the actual clinical experience both in Europe and in the United States. The records of the numerous American and European fasting clinics prove the truthfulness of the statement by Dr. Adolph Mayer, that "fasting is the most efficient means of correcting any disease". Fasting is, indeed, in the words of Dr. Otto H. F. Buchinger, Jr., M.D., a "Royal Road to Healing".

Fasting has been used throughout history, and is used quite extensively now, not only for the therapeutic purpose of healing disease, but also for its obvious rejuvenating and revitalizing effect. Thousands of people throughout the world fast regularly not to cure any particular disease, but because they consider fasting to be an effective way to cleanse the body from accumulated wastes, build up the physical stamina and the resistance against diseases, and revitalize and rejuvenate the functions of all their vital organs. Particularly in Sweden fasting has become a new national sport. This is done in groups and individually, mostly without medical supervision, but sometimes at the numerous health spas. The objective of these fasts is the periodic body cleansing and total rejuvenation of all the functions of the body.

Contrary to the popular notion, *you don't get weakened or depleted by fasting;* the opposite is true. After fasting you will feel stronger and revitalized; your health condition will be markedly improved, your physical and mental working capacity greatly increased. You not only will feel revitalized but also will look younger than before fasting. And this is not only because of lost pounds, but mostly because fasting has such a profound rejuvenating effect on the functions of all the vital organs, including the functions of the all-important endocrine glands, which are so decidedly responsible for how young or how old you feel and look.

The remarkable case of Miss A. L.

I have supervised hundreds of fasts, and have fasted many times myself. I have seen many remarkable cases of the dramatic effect of fasting upon patients who were ill, as well as upon those who fasted primarily for the purpose of rejuvenating and revitalizing themselves. Here is one recent case to illustrate the point.

Miss A.L. came to our Spa in a rather desperate condition. She had been working most of her life in the field of health and beauty. She had operated a figure control salon in Los Angeles and helped countless women and men to better health and better figures through proper exercises, plus a gym-type program of steam baths, swimming and workouts. For years she had been a wonderful advertisement for the effectiveness of her methods. But, as a conventional saying goes, all good things must come to an end. Time caught up with her. When she reached 45 her health and her looks started to deteriorate. She began putting on weight and, in spite of her rigid program of exercises, didn't seem to be able to control it. The signs of premature aging appeared suddenly. Her hair started to turn gray. Wrinkles appeared on her face. In addition, she felt stiffness and pain in her fingers, elbows and shoulders, which was diagnosed by her doctor as early symptoms of rheumatoid arthritis. Also, her complexion began to deteriorate rapidly. Her skin was dry and lifeless, and patches of psoriasis appeared behind her ears. She felt exhausted most of the time and lost interest in her work. She sold her business and tried to find new interests – without success.

In the meantime she developed an uncontrollable appetite and was putting on pounds each week. She had always wanted to work with young people and tried to get a job as a health, beauty and personality counselor in a home for young girls, but was turned down because of her "age and overweight". This incident was a great shock to her and a turning point in her life. She suddenly realized that she had to do something, and do it fast, if she didn't want to live the rest of her life in her words "as a fat, old, sick blob."

She had noticed with a horror that people started to feel sorry for her and that some of her former friends started to avoid her. Her personality had changed. Her outlook on life was negative. She had grown critical of everyone and everything, and her temper was getting worse and worse. No wonder her circle of friends was steadily diminishing.

There are hundreds of thousands of women who are in a similar situation. They blame their "condition" on the "change of life" and usually become resigned to the idea that they are becoming old and that nothing can be done about it. But Miss L. was not ready to give up. She decided to pull herself out of her dismal condition. Although working most of her life in a figure control and beauty field, she never thought much about nutrition and what role it plays in health. However, when some friends showed her my books and the advertisment for our health spa, she decided to make a visit and give it a try.

Miss L. was 54 when she came under my care, weighed 184 pounds and looked like 60. She told me frankly, that she didn't care much about arthritis, but that she had to improve her looks and her figure in order to "get that job" they refused her in Los Angeles. She was ready to do anything!

I outlined a three-month program for Miss L. First, one month of fasting on juices. Then a controlled raw food diet with special vitamins and mineral supplements for four weeks. After that two more weeks of fasting and two weeks of dieting. I promised that she would lose 50 pounds and look more like 40 than 60.

Miss L. followed my program religiously. She received two glasses of diluted fruit juice, one glass of vegetable juice, one glass of vegetable broth, and two cups of herb tea each day.* In addition, she could drink any amount of plain water she wanted. She took long walks, up to five miles a day. She was advised to take enemas twice a day. For arthritis, she followed a special program of biological treatments with dry brush massage, hot and cold showers, special exercises, castor oil packs, and thermal baths. All symptoms of her arthritis disappeared completely by the end of the first 30 day fast. And she had lost 28 pounds.

She lost an additional 12 pounds during the 30 days of raw-food diet. She ate three meals of the most delicious raw vegetables and tropical fruits each day in addition to the regular juices. She also took lecithin, kelp, Brewer's yeast and vitamins B, C, A and E. During an additional two weeks of fasting Miss A. L. lost 12 more pounds. By the end of three months, she had a total weight loss of 52 pounds.

When she left the spa, Miss A. L. weighted 132 pounds. From size 20, she had reduced to size 12, and had to shop for some new clothes before she could return to Los Angeles. She could neither feel nor see any traces of arthritis whatsoever. And the psoriasis patches behind her ears had vanished, too.

But you should have seen the change in her looks and her personality! From being an old, tired, apathetic, discouraged and disillusioned woman three months earlier, Miss L. now looked like a young woman of 40, filled with energy and enthusiasm, full of exciting plans for the future, determined to "get that job" she had been refused. Her vitality and enthusiasm were limitless and the change in her appearance was nothing but miraculous.

When she first began fasting, she was worried that if she lost all of that fat, her skin would be looser and flabbier, and she would look even more wrinkled. I assured her that with this kind of scientific juice fasting and the intermittent diet of vital foods and vitamin supplements, in conjunction with special exercises and dry brush massage, her system would be supplied with all the elements necessary for the effective regeneration and revitaliza-

---

*See the next chapter for detailed fasting program and the recipe for vegetable broth.

tion of her glandular activity and skin activity. Her collagen* – the deterioration of which is mainly responsible for premature wrinkles – would be strengthened and its elasticity restored; her new-cell building and cell repair accelerated; her muscle tone improved; her complexion receive new life. She was amazed at the fact that although she had lost so much weight in such a short time, her skin *was* tighter than before, her wrinkles *were* less noticeable and her previously muddy and gray complexion *had* acquired a fresh, radiant look.

Why fasting is the number one healer and rejuvenator

As I suggested before, the main causes of disease and aging are to be found in the processes of cell metabolism and cell regeneration.

First, as the famous Canadian "stress doctor", Hans Selye, said, "Life, the biological chain that holds our parts together, is only as strong as its weakest vital link." **You are as young or as old as your smallest vital links – the cells. The aging begins when your normal process of cell regeneration and rebuilding slows down. This slowdown is caused mainly by the accumulation of waste products in the tissues which interferes with the nourishment of the cells. Each cell of your body is a complete living entity with its own metabolism – it needs a constant supply of oxygen and sufficient nourishment in the form of all the known nutritive substances. When due to nutritional deficiencies, sluggish metabolism, sedentary life, overeating and consequent poor digestion and assimilation of food, lack of fresh air and sufficient exercise and rest, our cells are deprived of the nourishment they need, they start to degenerate and break down, the normal process of cell replacement and rebuilding slows down and your body starts to grow old, its resistance to diseases will diminish and various ills

---

*Collagen – intercellular substance that holds cells together, even the cells of the skin.

**Hans Selye, M.D., THE STRESS OF LIFE, McGraw-Hill Book Co., Inc. New York, 1956.

will start to appear. This may happen at any age. Sluggish metabolism, constipation, and consequent inefficient elimination causes retention and accumulation of toxic wastes in the tissues which interfere with the nourishment of the cells, causing disease and premature aging.

Second, only about half of your cells are in the peak of development, vitality, and working condition. One fourth are usually in the process of development and growth and the other fourth in the process of dying and replacement. The healthy vital life-processes and perpetual youth are maintained when there is perfect balance in this process of cell break-down and replacement. If the cells are breaking down and dying at a faster rate than the new cells are built, the process of aging will begin to set in. Also, it is of vital importance that the aging and the dying cells are decomposed and eliminated from the system as efficiently as possible. Quick and effective elimination of dead cells stimulates the building and growth of new cells.

Here's where fasting comes in as the most effective way to restore your health and rejuvenate your body. During the fast the process of elimination of the dead and dying cells is speeded up, the new-building of cells is accelerated and stimulated. At the same time the toxic waste products that interfere with the nourishment of the cells are effectively eliminated and the normal metabolic rate and cell oxygenation are restored.

How can the mere abstinence from food accomplish such remarkable results? Here's how:

1. During a prolonged fast (after the first three days), your body will live on its own substance. When it is deprived of the needed nutrition, your body will burn and digest its own tissues by the process of *autolysis,* or self-digestion. But your body will not do it indiscriminately! In its wisdom – and here lies the secret of the extraordinary effectiveness of fasting as curative and rejuvenating therapy! – your body will first decompose and burn those cells and tissues which are diseased, damaged, aging or dead. In fasting, your body feeds itself on the most impure and inferior materials, such as dead cells and morbid accumulations, tumors,

abcesses, damaged tissues, fat deposits, etc. Dr. Buchinger Sr., one of the greatest fasting authorities in the world, calls fasting – very pertinently – a "refuse disposal", a "burning of rubbish". These dead cells and inferior tissues are consumed and utilized *first.* The essential tissues and vital organs, the glands, the nervous system and the brain, are spared.

2. During fasting, while the old cells and diseased tissues are decomposed and burned, the building of new, healthy cells is stimulated and speeded up. This may seem unbelievable, since no nourishment, or only a limited amount of nourishment (during a juice fast), is supplied. But it is nevertheless a physiological fact. During the famous Swedish fast marches it was observed that the protein level of the blood (serum albumin reading) of fasting people remained constant and normal throughout the fasting period, *in spite of the fact that no protein was consumed.* The reason for this is that proteins in your body are in the so-called dynamic state; that is, they are changed from one stage to another, being decomposed and resynthesized constantly and re-used for various needs within the body. Amino acids, the building blocks of proteins, are not wasted, but are released from the decomposed cells and used again in the new-building of young, vital cells. As you know, your cells are made mostly of proteins and the complete set of all the essential amino acids is needed for the effective building of cells. During fasting the proteins needed for new cell building are resynthesized from the decomposed cells. Thus the body is using and re-using the same proteins and other nutrients over and over where they are needed.

3. During a fast, the eliminative and cleansing capacity of the eliminative organs – lungs, liver, kidneys, and skin – is greatly increased, and masses of accumulated metabolic wastes and toxins are quickly expelled. For example, during fasting the concentration of toxins in the urine can be ten times higher than normal. This is due to the fact that the eliminative organs are relieved from the usual burden of digesting foods and eliminating the resultant wastes, and can concentrate on the cleansing of old, accumulated wastes and toxins such as uric acid, purines, etc. from the tissues.

This eliminative process is evidenced by the following typical symptoms of fasting: offensive breath, dark urine, continuous and generous discharge from the colon with enema, skin eruptions, perspiration, catarrhal elimination of mucus, etc. Keep in mind that the activity of the human bowel system is not limited to the absorption of nutrients from the foods and the elimination of the undigestable food residues. Bowels are also one of your eliminative and detoxifying organs in a general sense: through the intestinal walls the toxins and metabolic wastes from the blood and tissues are discharged into the intestinal canal to be excreted from the body. This internal excretion is accelerated during fasting.

4. A fast affords a physiological rest to the disgestive, assimilative and protective organs of the body. After fasting, the digestion of food and the utilization of nutrients is greatly improved, and sluggishness and further waste retention is prevented. The rejuvenated cells are thus supplied with nutrients and oxygen more effectively.

5. Finally, the fast exerts a normalizing, stabilizing and rejuvenating effect on all the vital physiological, nervous and mental functions. The nervous system is rejuvenated; mental powers are improved; glandular chemistry and hormonal secretions are stimulated; biochemical and mineral balance in the tissues is normalized.

It is easy to see from the above why fasting is such an effective health-restoring and rejuvenating measure.

A few actual cases of successful fasting

Here, in a nutshell, are just a few cases of fasts I supervised in Canada, Mexico and Europe to illustrate the effectiveness, and the broad range of application, of this *the most effective healing method known to man.*

Mr. C. H. 72. ARTHRITIS IN KNEES AND SPINE, NEURITIS IN LEGS, EMPHYSEMA

When Mr. H. arrived at our Spa, he used a cane and could walk only a few yards with great difficulty. He had had arthritis for 35 years and underwent cortisone treatment 10 years previously. Due to severe painful neuritis in his legs below the knees, his nights were often sleepless. Only heavy doses of a codeine-containing drug made sleep possible. Even the slightest exertion caused shortness of breath due to his emphysema. He could not benefit from our thermal mineral baths and sauna because they were located 400 yards down a steep hill.

The day we began the biological program with a two week fast, Mr. H. asked me:

"I sure wish I could get down to the hot river and the baths. Do you think I will ever be able to do that?"

"In a month or so you'll be hopping like a goat around here, even down to the river," I promised him optimistically, concealing as well as I could my own doubts that such improvement could come so quickly, seeing how incapacitated he was.

In less than three weeks Mr. H. was walking without his cane and one day he reported to me triumphantly that he had walked to the baths and up the hill all by himself – without his cane! After two two-week fasts on juices, herb teas and vegetable broth, with an intermediate special arthritic diet* including *vitamin and mineral supplements,* plus special packs, hot and cold showers, dry brush massage and a series of special exercises, Mr. H. told me one day that he walked over two miles up and down the steep hills and along the river and "without any pain in his knees or shortness of breath!"

"It's great! I can't believe it," said Mr. H. gratefully.

MR. W. K., 58, ANGINA, CHRONIC LOW BACK PAIN, HIGH BLOOD PRESSURE

A typical American business executive, Mr. K., took two weeks off his busy schedule to come to our Spa demonstrating that he was, after all, not really "typical." The typical American businessman works himself up to his heart attack and premature

---

*Outlined in detail in THERE IS A CURE FOR ARTHRITIS, Parker Publishing Co., West Nyack, N.Y. 1968.

death trying to make his first million, never permitting himself time for a holiday or a trip to a health Spa.

Mr. K. had blood pressure of 160/90, severe angina pains in the chest and a shortness of breath. He also had an arthritic condition in the lumbar region of his spine and several large fatty tumors in his body, one of the size of an egg on his right forearm.

After ten days of fasting on juices and vegetable broths and 4 days of breaking the fast on a raw vegetable and fruit diet, his blood pressure went down to 115/70; arthritic pain in the lower back almost completely disappeared ("90% better," he told me); he could walk for miles each day without chest pain or breathing difficulties; and his fatty tumor on the right arm was reduced to the size of an almond. It would probably have disappeared completely if Mr. K. had had the opportunity to stay a couple of more weeks.

MRS. A. J., 64, HIGH BLOOD PRESSURE, IRREGULAR HEART BEAT, CHRONIC HEADACHES

After seven days of juice fasting, Mrs. J.'s blood pressure went from 160/100 to 135/80. Headaches disappeared as if by a miracle. She continued on a special salt-free diet of raw foods with lots of garlic, comfrey, and special vitamin supplements of E, C, and B-complex, with B_{15}. Her heart functioning improved considerably, and the blood pressure remained normal when checked three weeks later.

MISS C. F., 28, ASTHMA

Miss F. suffered from one of the most severe cases of asthma I have seen. She had been totally dependent on a heavy dosage of drugs for over 10 years.

I suggested a fast on diluted juices for a week, to be followed by a strictly raw food diet, with a teaspoonful of plain lemon juice before each meal, several comfrey leaves chewed raw, and several cloves of garlic each day.

After one week of fasting, Miss F. felt so much better that she actually begged me to let her continue another week. At the end of the second week she still didn't have any desire to quit fasting.

"I feel so good, with much less frequent attacks, that I want to continue fasting for one more week," she said.

After 3 weeks of fasting she finally broke the fast and started with a special diet and vitamin supplements. She took 1,200 I.U. of E each day, 3,000 mg. of vitamin C, and 50 mg. of B_{15}. In addition she received B-complex, brewer's yeast, mineral supplements, lecithin, kelp and whey. She also took special breathing exercises, dry brush massage, and hot and cold showers in the morning.

She left the Spa so much improved that her medication was reduced by two thirds after 10 years of constant use. Her breathing was dramatically improved and her vitality and strength greatly increased. She could now walk long distances without any discomfort or shortness of breath.

MRS. L. K., 54, CHRONIC BRONCHITIS, CHRONIC TONSILITIS, HIGH BLOOD PRESSURE

Mrs. K. had blood pressure of 150/90. She was overweight and troubled by chronic colds and chronic bronchial catarrh for over 10 years, with cough and a voluminous discharge of mucus.

In two weeks of juice fasting, she reduced 12 pounds, her blood pressure went down to 128/78, and her chronic bronchitis and tonsilitis were completely cleared up – no cough, no mucus, no breathing discomfort.

MISS A. Y., 48, ARTHRITIS, OVERWEIGHT, PSORIASIS

Miss A. undertook a long fast of 28 days. She used vegetable broth morning and night, diluted vegetable juices at 1:00 and

6:00 P.M. and diluted fruit juices (no citrus) at 10:00 A.M. and 4:00 P.M. She took enemas twice a day, hot and cold showers, and dry brush massage. She walked and exercised every day.

As her fasting progressed, Miss A. became more and more enthusiastic about the anticipated results. Instead of becoming weaker, she felt stronger with each passing day. She started with short walks, because of arthritis in her knees, but gradually increased the distance, until she walked about 5 miles each day.

Her arthritis, both swelling and pain, completely disappeared after the first 2 weeks. Psoriasis patches decreased in size gradually and after 4 weeks of fasting were completely gone. She reduced 25 pounds and looked not only healthier, but also at least 10 years younger.

Fasting, vitality and sex

Those who have never tried fasting and are not familiar with the physiology of fasting, usually think that fasting will make them weak. The amazing fact about juice fasting, which shocks and pleasantly surprises practically all those who fast for the first time, is that fasting actually makes them stronger and increases their vitality. During the first few days of the fast, the patient feels hungry and somewhat weak, but after the third day the hunger usually disappears, and vitality and strength begins to increase with every fasting day. We advise fasters to continue with their usual work, if they are fasting at home, or to do lots of exercise and walking if they are fasting under supervision at a spa. Our patients usually walk long distances, some as much as 5 to 10 miles a day. Walking in the open is the best and most beneficial form of exercise for any age or any condition as well as the best way to prevent disease.

I have made a remarkable observation during many years of supervising fasts. Many men have reported that they have experienced a renewed sexual vigor after 7, 10 or more days of fasting.

One man, age 62, who felt his sexual life had been very inadequate for a long time, told me that on the 8th day of fasting he suddenly felt such a sex urge that he was not able to refrain from sexual intercourse. He was somewhat reluctant because he certainly didn't expect "this sort of thing" during the fast. His wife told him, "Darling, you should fast more often!"

Another striking case was that of Dr. N.D., who was 78 years old and fasted under my supervision for his arthritis. He told me after 6 days of fasting:

"A most extraordinary thing happened yesterday! I had a most wonderful sex affair with my wife. For the last 7 or 8 years, my sex life was rather sporadic; and in the last 6 months or so I had nothing but the sweet memories of the past. But yesterday . . . How can you explain that?"

I can explain "that". A life-long sexual virility is every man's birthright. "Bedroom fatigue" is not caused by old age, but by neglected, malnourished and atrophied endocrine glands, which are responsible for deteriotating physical and sexual vitality. Premature signs of aging, loss of interest in sex, bulging waistline – all these are signs of insufficiently functioning endocrine or sex glands and diminished sex hormone production. Fasting has an energizing, invigorating effect on the activity and functions of all organs and glands, including the functions of the endocrine glands. I have heard many reports of the rejuvenating and revitalizing effect of fasting on sexual vigor and ability.

Sex urge is motivated by extra, surplus energy. A sick man is a poor lover. All his energy goes on trying to keep going, fighting chronic fatigue and pain. The ill man has no surplus energy left for sex. Fasting restores health, normalizes all the body functions, wipes out pain and gives a new vitality and energy surplus. The renewed sexual drive is one of the surest indications that the health and strength have returned.

Is fasting safe?

The examples cited earlier in this chapter show how safe fasting is. Fasting up to 40 days on water and up to 100 days, or even longer, on juices, is considered perfectly safe. In the Swedish hospital experiments, patients fasted 55 days without any apparent harm. I know of a perfectly healthy young man of 27, who fasted 143 days; not for any particular disease, but to cleanse, regenerate and rejuvenate his body and mind. One Scottish woman, mentioned before, fasted 249 days on juices and not only did she not harm herself, but she improved her looks and her health considerably. In European clinics thousands of patients have fasted up to 40 days. And the Swedish fast marches demonstrated very dramatically the safety of fasting, even during adverse conditions of severe stress.

The truth is that *fasting is one of the safest healing methods known to medical science.* As a matter of fact, you can live without food for months, but can kill yourself by overeating in a few weeks. Nobody ever died of a few weeks of *intentional* fasting. During *involuntary,* prolonged starvation, the negative state of mind and fear for life exert a paralyzing, disruptive and destructive effect on all the body functions, and will cause both physical damage and eventual death. Only during *intentional* fasting, when you have complete understanding, confidence and faith in the constructive, beneficial effect of fasting, will your body initiate its health-restoring and regenerative processes and receive nothing but a beneficial effect.

Naturally, if you suffer from a serious condition such as cancer, diabetes, tuberculosis, cardio-vascular disorder, or any other serious disease, you should be at all times under a doctor's supervision. Although juice fasting up to 10 days or two weeks is not a dangerous measure and could be undertaken at home and without supervision, my advice is that if you do not have a thorough understanding and insight into all phases and details of fasting, you should try to find an experienced practitioner who will supervise your fast. This will give you peace of mind and confidence in the treatment, which are imperative for the successful outcome of any therapeutic measure. The cleansing and health-restoring activity of fasting will bring about many physiological changes in your body. These changes may manifest themselves in certain discomforts, or what is called fasting crises, such as headache, coated tongue, foul breath, dizziness, skin eruption, and even temporary worsening of the condition. When fasting is supervised by an experienced practitioner, he will assure you that these reactions should give you no cause for concern, they are common symptoms of fasting, and properly understood, should not discourage you from continuing with the fast.

What about fasting and DDT?

It has been suggested by some writers recently that because of the universal poisoning by DDT, fasting can be dangerous. DDT, to which we all are exposed these days through insecticide contaminated foods, is a cumulative poison which is stored in the fat tissues of the body. During fasting, when the body starts to feed itself on its own tissues, fat is broken down and digested, releasing dangerous amounts of DDT into the blood stream. This can cause symptoms of acute DDT poisoning.

The danger of DDT poisoning during reducing regimes or fasting, due to the rapid break down of fat tissues, has been known for a long time. The way fasting is administered in some American clinics – a total water fast without enema and staying in bed – a sudden DDT release can be dangerous. When fasting is done correctly, however, the danger is minimal. If you fast according to the recommendations of this book on fresh fruit and vegetable juices and vegetable broth, plenty of exercise and daily enemas – you are well protected from any real danger in this respect. First, DDT is released into the blood stream more slowly than in a total water fast; and, second, DDT and other poisons are better neutralized and more efficiently and safely excreted from the body because of the rich mineral and vitamin content of the juices and broth, particularly the vitamin C, calcium and potassium.. Daily enemas, the extensive program of revitalizing skin activity, lots of walking and deep breathing, and the medicinal, protective effect of raw fruits and vegetable juices, broths, and herb teas – all these help to make your fasting perfectly safe, even in respect to the release of DDT into the bloodstream. It would be advisable, however, that if you are quite overweight, and want to fast strictly for reducing, you should go on a series of short fasts (one week or 10 day fasts) instead of one very long fast. This way the fat tissues will be burned at a slower rate, and toxins released at intervals and eliminated from your system more safely. Also, the addition of high doses of certain vitamins and food supplements, especially vitamin C, to the diet between fasts will help to protect your body from the harmful effects of toxic substances.

How long can you fast?

If fasting is undertaken for *prophylactic* purposes, that is to cleanse, regenerate and rejuvenate the body, one week or 10 days of fasting will be sufficient. Such short fasts can be taken once or twice a year. The length of the *therapeutic* fast, or fast undertaken with the purpose of healing, should be determined by the doctor or practitioner, who supervises the fast. The length of therapeutic fasts varies between 7 days and 40 days. The most common length of fasts in European clinics is 14 to 21 days. It would not be advisable to undertake a do-it-yourself fasting program for longer than one week or ten days. But if you have a proper mental attitude, confidence and understanding of the philosophy and physiology of fasting, you can safely fast on your own up to 10 days. Remember, you are not the first to try it – millions of people have done it successfully before you. I know you will be surprised and amazed both at the safety and the miraculous health-restoring and rejuvenating effect of fasting.

Chapter 9

How To Fast and How Not To

The classic form of fasting is a pure water fast – the abstinance from all foods and drinks with the exception of pure water. The renaissance of water fasting in the United States happened around the turn of the century. It was popularized here mainly by immigrant European nature-cure practitioners.

While in the last few decades the fasting methods in Europe have completely changed – and now practically all European clinics use exclusively juice fasting – most American practitioners and clinics specializing in fasting still use the antiquated water fast method. I have supervised both types of fasting and am thoroughly convinced of the superiority of juice fasting. Dr. Otto H. F. Buchinger, who has supervised more fasts than any other doctor (over 80,000 fasts), employs only juice fasting. He told me that, in his experience, fasting on the fresh raw juices of fruits and vegetables, plus vegetable broths and herb teas, results in much faster recovery from disease and more effective cleansing and rejuvenation of the tissues than does the traditional water fast.

Why juice fasting?

The medical justification of juice fasting is based on the following physiological facts:

- Raw juices, as well as freshly made vegetable broths, are rich in vitamins, minerals, trace elements and enzymes.
- These vital elements are very easily assimilated directly into the bloodstream, without putting a strain on the digestive system – thus they do not disrupt the healing and rejuvenating process of autolysis, or self-digestion, as suggested by some water fast proponents.
- Contrary to the opinion of some writers, fruit and vegetable juices do not stimulate the secretion of hydrochloric acid in the stomach, which can lead to ulcers. Hydrochloric acid is mainly secreted when protein-rich foods are eaten.
- The nutritive elements from the juices are extremely beneficial in normalizing all the body processes, supplying needed elements for the body's own healing activity and cell regeneration, and, thus, speeding recovery.
- Raw juices and vegetable broths provide an alkaline surplus which is extremely important for the proper acid-alkaline balance in the blood and tissues, since blood and tissues contain large amounts of acids during fasting.
- Generous amounts of minerals in the juices, particularly in the vegetable broth, help to restore the biochemical and mineral balance in the tissues and cells. Mineral imbalance in the tissues is one of the main causes of diminished oxygenation, which leads to disease and the premature aging of cells.
- According to Dr. Ralph Bircher, raw juices contain an as yet unidentified factor which stimulates what he calls a micro-electric tension in the body and is responsible for the cells' ability to absorb nutrients from the bloodstream and effectively excrete metabolic wastes.

Thus, raw juice fasting is of particular importance when you fast for regeneration and rejuvenation of your body. Juice fasting will help to break down and dispose of the old dying cells, revitalize the active cells, and accelerate the new-building of young, vital cells.

Are you fasting or not?

The proponents of water fast like to tell you that the juice fast is *not* a fast, it is a *liquid diet.* They misunderstand the therapeutic meaning of fasting. *Any condition when your body is encouraged to initiate the process of autolysis, or self-digestion, is fasting.* During juice fasting, when no solid foods, proteins or fats are consumed, your body will decompose and burn all the diseased and inferior protein and fat tissues, just as it does during the water fast. Juices are absorbed directly into the bloodstream without the usual process of digestion. The only difference between the juice fast and the water fast is that during the juice fast your body's eliminative and detoxifying capacity is increased; the healing processes are speeded up and you feel less debilitated. But if someone insists upon calling this superior healing method a *juice diet,* instead of a *juice fast,* let him do it if it makes him happy!

Should you take enemas?

There is a great deal of controversy on the advisability of enemas during fasting. There are some practitioners in the United States who condemn the use of enemas or colonic irrigations completely. They claim that enemas are unnecessary, unnatural, harmful and habit-forming. In their writings, the "anti-enemists" love to retort with the argument, "Animals do not take enemas when they fast. Why should man?"

How could one respond to the above fatuous reasoning except by saying that animals do not write books, give health lectures or engage in medical research either! In all fairness, however, it must be said that "anti-chemists" are right in saying that enemas are unnatural and habit-forming. As a rule, enemas should not be used regularly or for prolonged periods, as, for example, a regular routine to cope with chronic constipation. The emptying of your bowel is accomplished "naturally" by regular muscle contractions in the intestines, called peristalsis. These contractions are started in healthy individuals by the special defecation-reflex which is triggered by pressure from the filled rectum. The enema fills the rectum with water, and causes the artificial, strong pressure that triggers the defecation mechanism. If used regularly, enemas, with their instant and powerful pressure, will weaken the natural sensitivity of the mechanism; after a while, it will not readily respond to the more subtle, natural stimulus. Therefore, those who make a daily habit of using enemas will find that their bowels have lost the natural ability to empty the wastes. Thus, enemas used regularly can be considered habit-forming.

However, the above reasoning has nothing to do with the *use of enemas during fasting.* While virtually all European fasting specialists warn against the regular use of enemas and colonics, they *all agree* that there are some important exceptions to this rule. The most notable of these is fasting. (The other conditions where an enema is advised are acute constipation and acute infectious diseases, and when the patient is bedridden for prolonged periods, which, because of total lack of motion, causes sluggishness in normal bowel movements.)

During fasting, the natural stimulation of the defecation-reflex from food is missing and therefore all the impurities, wastes and toxins will remain in the body and may cause auto-toxemia, or self-poisoning. The main purpose of fasting is to help the body to cleanse itself from accumulated toxic wastes. By the process of autolysis, a huge amount of morbid matter, dead cells and diseased tissues are burned; and the toxic wastes which have accumulated in the tissues for years, causing disease and premature aging, are loosened and expelled from the system. The alimentary canal, the digestive and eliminative system, is the main road by which these toxins are thrown out of the body. Since, during fasting, the natural bowel movements cease to take place, the toxic wastes would have no way of leaving the system, except with the help of enemas.

This is why virtually all biological doctors in Europe administer enemas to all fasting patients – once, twice and some even three times a day. *Enemas during fasting will assist the body in its cleansing and detoxifying effort by washing out all the toxic wastes from the alimentary canal.*

Constipation is one of the most common ailments of civilized man. As a consequence of long-standing constipation, the digestive tract, particularly in the lower bowels and colon, becomes slack and stagnant with hardened residues clinging to the walls of the colon and filling its many pockets and folds. This results in putrefaction and gas, forming a source of slow poisoning of the whole body. Diverticulitis, a chronic condition where small pouches and pockets of the colon are packed with feces, is one of the most common complaints of most people over 50, particularly women. Often the whole length of the colon is completely packed with old, hardened fecal matter, cemented to the walls and pockets, leaving only a thin, narrow channel which enables soft feces to pass through. To let the patients fast without making an effort to wash out this constant source of auto-intoxication, is indeed unwise. During fasting, copious amounts of toxins are released from the tissues and thrown into the bloodstream for elimination. If these toxins can not come out through the alimentary canal, the body will try to get them out through other eliminative organs, particularly through the kidneys, which, as a result, will often be overloaded and even damaged.

All our fasting patients are given daily enemas in addition to colonic irrigations once a week. To further assist the body in its detoxification and elimination processes, fasting patients are given dry brush massage twice a day to stimulate the eliminative capacity of the skin, the biggest eliminative organ*. Patients are also advised to walk and exercise in fresh air as much as possible to help the lungs in their blood-purification work.

---

*See next chapter.

Fasting without enemas can be harmful

I have seen rather horrifying examples of what prolonged water fasting without enemas can do. A few months ago, a man arrived at our Spa from recent treatments at a famous American clinic where he fasted for 32 days on water. During all this time he was advised to stay in bed. He was given no enemas or colonic irrigations. He told me that it took him two months "to recuperate" from this fast and get on his feet. He was still in a very weak condition with damaged kidneys and severe edema in his legs. Several former patients of this particular clinic advised me that they were told at the clinic that it takes an amount of time equal to the fasting time to recuperate from the effects of fasting. That is, one month of fasting will require one month of recuperating time. When this man told me of his experience, I showed him one of my patients, who was just completing the last day of his one-month juice fast. He was active all the time during fasting, walked 3 to 5 miles each day, took yoga and other exercises, *had enemas twice a day,* and felt on the last day of the fast stronger and healthier than before the fast. He was actually loaded with vitality. This patient did not need any recuperating period *after* his fast – *his fast indeed was a recuperative and regenerative period!*

Of course, fasting is such a miraculous healing measure that even fasting on water and *without* enemas accomplishes some good in many cases. But how much better results the fasting would accomplish *with* the enema and the addition of raw juices!

How to take an enema

To take an enema, you must have an enema can or bag with a rubber hose and a nozzle; it can be obtained at any drug store.

Fill the enema bag with lukewarm water, about 99 degrees F. Add a few drops of fresh lemon juice, or a cup of camomile tea (can be bought at health food stores); however, the enema can be taken with plain water. For a do-it-yourself enema, 1 pint to 1 quart of water is sufficient.

The best position for taking an enema is on your knees, head down to the floor, with enema bag hanging 2½ to 3 feet above the anus, to get sufficient pressure in the flow of water. The flow can be regulated by squeezing the tube with the fingers; some enema bags have a special clamp to regulate the flow. Before inserting the nozzle into the anus make sure there is no air left in the tube; let water run out for a moment. Use some vaseline, oil or other lubricator on the nozzle to make insertion easier. If you feel discomfort or pain when water is running in, stop the flow for a while and take deep breaths, then continue again until the bag is empty.

If you can retain the water for a while and do not feel forced to empty the bowels at once, you may lie on a bed or soft rug for a few minutes, and let the water do its dissolving and washing work before letting it out. First lie on the back for a minute, then on the right side, then on the stomach and then on the left side. While you are doing this, gently massage your stomach with your hands. Then go to the toilet and let the water run out. Stay long enough to make sure that the bowels are empty.

The enema should be taken at least once each fasting day. The best time is the first thing in the morning. After the fast is broken, enemas should be continued until the bowels begin to move naturally without the help of the enemas. This usually takes two or three days. As soon as normal peristalsis is established, enemas should be discontinued.

Here are some additional points to watch:

- Make sure that the enema water is not too cold or too hot; it should be of body temperature, or slightly above.
- Keep the equipment clean; wash it with soap and water. If several people use the equipment, disinfect the nozzle with rubbing alcohol, then rinse with water.
- And finally, watch for the copious amounts of debris and ill-smelling wastes coming out with the enema water, even after 5 weeks of fasting!

Note: the enemas are given in *all* European biological clinics that I am familiar with, and I am familiar with most of them.

But the number of enemas varies with various practitioners. At Buchinger Sanatorium, enemas are given once every morning or every second morning. At Sweden's Björkagården Institute, as well as at Dr. Lars-Erik Essén's Vita Nova (both presented in detail in my book *THERE IS A CURE FOR ARTHRITIS*), enemas are administered 2 or 3 times a day – morning, noon and evening. Some clinics give enemas twice a day. My own recommendation is at least once a day, taken each morning.

DETAILED PROGRAM FOR DO-IT-YOURSELF FASTING FOR BETTER HEALTH AND LONGER LIFE

It is advisable to prepare yourself for fasting by a short cleansing diet. For 2 or 3 days eat nothing but raw fruits and vegetables – one meal made of any available fruits, the other of fresh vegetable salad.

Fasting usually begins with an effective bowel cleansing with the help of purgatives, such as Glauber's salts or castor oil. Dr. Otto Buchinger uses an ounce and a half of Glauber's salts in one and a quarter pints of warm water on the morning of the first day of fasting. Since the Glauber's salt drink is not very tasty, it is usually followed by a glass of fruit juice. Glauber's salts will cause repeated and powerful evacuations and cleanse your bowels thoroughly. Some European clinics use castor oil for the same purpose. On the first day of fasting, one or two hours before an enema, two tablespoons of pure castor oil is taken in a glass of water to which the juice of half a lemon has been added. Of course, you can begin your fasting without a purgative, just by using a double enema. First take 1 pint of plain water and let it out. Then repeat with a full quart of water into which camomile tea or a few drops of lemon juice have been added.

The next day, and each following day of the fast, you follow this program:

UPON ARISING:	Enema
AFTER ENEMA:	Dry brush massage, followed by hot and cold shower. (See instructions in Chapter 10)
9:00 A.M.	Cup of herb tea – lukewarm, not hot. Health food stores carry a large assortment of herb teas. I recommend peppermint, camomile, or rose hips. See the instructions on the package for preparing the teas.
11:00 A.M.	A glass of freshly-pressed fruit juice, diluted fifty-fifty with water.
11:00 A.M. to 1:00 P.M.	Walk or mild exercise, or sunbathing, if the weather permits. (In our Spa, various baths, massages and other treatments are given at this time.)
1:00 P.M.	A glass of freshly made vegetable juice or a cup of vegetable broth*.
1:30 to 4:00 P.M.	Rest in bed.
4:00 P.M.	Cup of herb tea.
4:15 P.M. to 7:00 P.M.	Walk, therapeutic baths, exercises or other treatments.
7:00 P.M.	Glass of diluted vegetable or fruit juice, or cup of vegetable broth.

Drink plain lukewarm water, or mineral water, when thirsty. The total juice and broth volume during the day should be between 1 ½ pints and 1 ½ quarts. Never dilute fresh juices with vegetable broth, only with pure water. The total liquid intake should be approximately 6 to 8 glasses – but don't hesitate to drink more, if thirsty.

---

*See recipe and directions later in this chapter.

Again, I suggest that, if at all possible, have your fasting supervised by someone who is well initiated in it. Under expert supervision such a fast could be undertaken at home up to 30 days, if necessary. If you are ill, you should consult your doctor on advisability of fasting in your case. Show this chapter and the instructions to your own doctor and ask him to supervise your fasting and examine your condition as the fast progresses. Without expert supervision I would not advise fasting longer than one week to 10 days at a time. After a few weeks on a health-building diet (see Chapter 3), your fasting program may be repeated.

How fast is broken

Whether your fast will turn out to be a success or a failure will depend largely on how you break your fast. *Breaking a fast is the most significant phase of it. The beneficial effect of fasting could be totally undone if the fast is broken incorrectly!* As Dr. Otto F. H. Buchinger says: "Even a fool can fast, but *only a wise man knows how to break the fast properly and to build up properly after the fast!*"

The main rules for breaking the fast are:

1. *Do not overeat!*
2. *Eat slowly and chew your food extremely well*
3. *Take several days of gradual transition to the normal diet.*

First day: Eat one whole apple in the morning and a very *small* bowl of raw vegetable salad at lunch, in addition to the usual juice and broth menu.

Second day: Soaked prunes or figs (with the soaking water) for breakfast. Small bowl of fresh vegetable salad for lunch. Vegetable soup made without salt at dinner. Two apples eaten between meals. All this in addition to the usual juices and broths.

Third day: As second day, but add a small glass of yogurt and a few raw nuts for breakfast. Increase the salad portion at lunch, and add a boiled or baked potato. A slice of whole-grain bread with butter and a slice of cheese with soup at evening.

Fourth day: You may start eating normally, adhering to a cleansing macrobiotic diet outlined in Chapter 3 of this book. If you fasted longer than 10 days, the break-in period should be extended one day for every 4 days of fasting.

In order to benefit from fasting to the greatest possible extent it is of paramount importance that after fasting a build-up diet of vital natural foods be maintained. Follow the general diet outlined in Chapter 3 of this book. Such a diet will supply the healing and regenerative forces of your body with all the needed elements, so that the cleansing, regenerative, rejuvenative and healing processes initiated by the body during fasting can be continued.

But *first and foremost,* keep always in mind the first rule of breaking the fast: *do not overeat!* This rule also happens to be the *first rule* of keeping healthy and staying young longer.

What juices to use

All juices used during fasting should be made fresh just before drinking. In our Spa, various juices are prescribed individually, depending on the particular condition of the patient. For example, arthritics are not given citrus juices, except once or twice a week, the emphasis is instead on vegetable juices, particularly carrots, celery and alfalfa juices, and twice a day vegetable broths. In some other conditions, the emphasis is on fruit juices. Fruits and vegetables have a health-restorative, medicinal value and, prescribed individually, can be effectively used to speed the recovery. In my book, *HOW TO KEEP SLIM, HEALTHY AND YOUNG WITH JUICE FASTING,* I describe the medicinal properties of various juices and what juices to use for specific conditions.*

---

* Paavo O. Airola, HOW TO KEEP SLIM, HEALTHY AND YOUNG WITH JUICE FASTING, published by Health Plus, Publishers.

If you are in a relatively healthy condition and are fasting for the purpose of purifying and cleansing your body and rejuvenating and regenerating all its vital functions, then you can use the juice of any available fruits and vegetables. Fruit juices most frequently used are: apple, orange, grapefruit, lemon, grapes, pineapple, pear. In Mexican Spas, the juices of two tropical fruits, papaya and lima, are used frequently. The recommended vegetable juices are: carrot, celery, cabbage, beets, and, of course, last but not least, the green juice, a "chlorophyll drink" made from green leaves of alfalfa, comfrey, carrot tops, beet tops, parsley, wheat grass, and/or any other available edible greens.

How to make vegetable broth

Vegetable broth is one of the standard beverages during fasting in all biological clinics in Europe. Our fasting patients receive a large glass of vegetable broth first thing in the morning and before going to bed. It is a cleansing and alkalizing drink which supplies a great amount of vitamins and particularly minerals, which are so important for establishing and normalizing a proper chemical balance in the tissues during fasting. Vegetable broth is particularly rich in the mineral *potassium* which is of special importance in the treatment of rheumatic diseases and arthritis. Here's how you make it:

Vegetable Broth

2 large potatoes, unpeeled, chopped or sliced to approximately one-half-inch pieces
1 cup carrots, shredded or sliced
1 cup beets, shredded or sliced
1 cup celery, leaves and all, chopped to one-half-inch pieces
1 cup any other available vegetables: beet tops, turnips and turnip tops, parsley, cabbage or a little of everything.
However, a satisfactory broth can be made with only potatoes, beets, carrots, and celery, consisting of approximately 50% potatoes.

Use stainless steel, enameled or earthenware utensil. Fill it up with one and one-half quarts of water and slice the vegetables directly into the water to prevent oxidation. Cover and cook slowly for at least a half hour. Let stand for another half hour, strain, cool until warm and serve. If not used immediately, keep in refrigerator. Warm it up before serving.

"Excelsior"

"Excelsior" drink is a variation of vegetable broth especially for patients with constipation problems and those with stomach and bowel disorders. Flax seeds have a healing effect on the stomach and bowel linings as well as act as a natural, mild laxative. Bran supplies necessary bulk and stimulates normal peristalsis. "Excelsior" should be used after fasting at least for the first few days or weeks, until the normal peristaltic rhythm is established.

1 cup of vegetable broth, as above
1 tbsp. whole flaxseed
1 tbsp. raw wheat bran

Flaxseed and wheat bran can be bought at health food stores. Soak flaxseed and wheat bran in vegetable broth overnight. In the morning, stir well, warm up and drink – seeds and all. *Do not chew the flaxseeds, drink them whole.* Actually, it would be better not to *drink* excelsior, but *eat* it slowly with a spoon, without chewing, to effect proper salivation.

Other tips on fasting

1. *Work.* Should you discontinue with your work and rest or stay in bed while fasting? Not at all! On the contrary, staying in bed during fasting is definitely harmful. Your body needs lots of assistance in the form of fresh air, motion and exercise, in order to accomplish a thorough cleansing of the blood and tissues and to effectively regenerate and revitalize all the body functions. Therefore, patients in the fasting clinics are advised to do lots of walking and mild exercises, especially deep breathing

exercises, in addition to sunbathing. If you fast on your own, it is advisable to continue with your normal activities, but perhaps avoid *too* strenuous physical or mental work. But do not neglect your daily walks! Do deep breathing exercises while you walk.

2. *Baths.* It is generally believed that one-third of all body impurities and wastes are eliminated through the skin. Since the tissue cleansing and speedy elimination of toxic wastes is a prime purpose of fasting, it is important to keep the skin pores wide open and the elimination through the skin as efficient as possible. Daily showers, especially in conjunction with dry brush massage are recommended. If the heart and circulation are good (your doctor must determine this) then hot baths, steambaths (saunas) and hot-and-cold showers should be taken frequently. (See chapters on Water Cure and Over-heating baths in my book, HEALTH SECRETS FROM EUROPE.)

3. *Dry brush massage.* During fasting – in fact, during the whole period of biological treatment – all our patients are advised to take dry brush massage. This is a simple and easy method of rejuvenating and revitalizing your skin and of increasing its capacity to eliminate accumulated poisons. Dry brush massage is taken for about 10 to 15 minutes each morning before the hot-and-cold shower, and again before going to bed at night. See next chapter for the detailed description of dry brush massage – the million-dollar health and beauty secret.

4. *Contra-indications for fasting.* There are a few diseases and conditions where prolonged fasting is not advised. Such diseases are: advanced cases of tuberculosis; active malignancies; advanced diabetes; and extreme emaciation or wasting disease. Extremely emaciated patients should not fast longer than up to three days at a time, with intervals of a nourishing diet. Where there is serious acute disease, do not attempt fasting without consulting your doctor and abide by his decision on the advisability of undertaking a fast.

5. *Drugs and fasting.* As a rule, a *complete withdrawal* of all drugs is advised during a fast. However, in certain conditions when drugs have been used for a long time and a certain body

dependence built up, withdrawal of drugs should be gradual and the effect of withdrawal carefully supervised by a doctor. Insulin in diabetes, digitalis in heart disease, or cortisone in arthritis or other diseases – these and a few other drugs should never be withdrawn suddenly and completely, but gradually, by diminishing the dosage each day. This even applies to regular coffee, if the patient has, for example, a heart condition and has been a heavy coffee-addict for years.

6. *Vitamins.* Should you take vitamins while fasting? As you can see in Chapter 4, I am positively an advocate of taking vitamins and food supplements – for the healthy as well as for the sick – mainly because of our devitalized foods and toxic environment. Also, I use vitamins extensively, often in huge doses, in my therapeutic programs for practically any condition of ill health. But while fasting, the intake of vitamins or other food supplements should be discontinued completely. The general rule is that vitamin and mineral supplements should be taken only when food is eaten; they can be properly used by the body only in combination with foods.

However, as with drugs in certain conditions, there are cases when certain vitamins can be allowed while fasting. Serious heart cases, for example, are given vitamin E during the fast, although in diminished dosage. The doctor who supervises your fast must determine the necessity of continuing with vitamins while fasting.

As soon as fast is broken, from the second or third day, the usual vitamin supplementation can be resumed.

7. *Hunger.* Will you feel hungry during fasting? Yes, during the first three or four days you will feel hungry, of course. But after that the hunger usually disappears. As a matter of fact, the unbelievable will happen: the longer you fast the less hungry you feel. Finally, when the body has completed its cleansing and restorative work it will signal to you by a sudden and definite feeling of hunger that you should start eating. *This is physiologically the right time to break the fast.* Of course, in the case of juice fasts, even during the first three or four days you will hardly

feel any hunger at all. However, every patient reacts differently in this respect; much of it depends on the mental attitude. Those who are not totally convinced of the positive properties of fasting, or if they fast unwillingly (nobody should fast unwillingly!), they will feel more hungry than those who have complete faith and confidence in fasting. The amount of will power and determination plays an important role, too. Some of our fasting patients come to the dining room where a smorgasbord table, loaded with most appetizing dishes, tempts them, and drink their water or juice without being tempted in the least. Others beg me every day to let them start eating, although all symptoms indicate that they have no real physiological appetite. This difference in the personality make-up is one good reason why the best way to fast is at a fasting clinic or health Spa where the practitioner can closely observe the patient, encourage him to continue, and explain his various reactions and symptoms, and where fasting guests can encourage one another.

8. *Mental attitude.* Mental attitude during fasting is of paramount importance. Avoid negative influences. Do not listen to terrified relatives and "friends" who will warn you that you will pass out any moment. As I said before, nobody has ever died as a result of a few weeks of intentional fasting. Have confidence in what you are doing. Remember, you are not the first to try it – millions of people have done it successfully before you. If it makes you feel better, do not call this measure a fast call it a liquid diet.

It is best not to tell your friends of your new exciting venture. If they know you are fasting, they will study you carefully and tell you how much worse you look each day. If they don't know of your fasting, they will ask you, "What's happening, you look better and better each day?" Such is human nature! I know from a quarter of a century of experience that when your fast is over, both you and your friends will be surprised and amazed at the remarkable – yes, miraculous – transformation that has taken place.

9. *Fasting and spiritual awareness.* Fasting not only accomplishes a physiological regeneration and revitalization of your body, but has a profound stimulating effect on your mental faculties. It also increases your spiritual awareness. It is important, therefore, to adopt a proper, relaxed attitude. Try to disassociate yourself from the usual everyday problems and the worries of the material world, and let the refinement and perfection of your inner self come to the fore as the ultimate purpose of your existence.

Fasting is the time of rest, meditation and renewal of body, mind and spirit. In all religions – Oriental, Hebrew, Christian, Muhammadan – periodic fasting played a vital part, for two reasons: *one,* to keep the body (the temple of the spirit) clean; *two,* to keep the spirit attuned with its Divine source.

You will notice that during fasting your visual and mental perception and awareness of aesthetic beauty will be sharpened and that your thoughts will gradually raise from a lower, everyday level of unpleasant realities to higher realities, concerned with the purpose and meaning of your Divinely designed life. Your daily walk in the woods will be a new and totally different experience. The singing of the birds will sound like the most inspiring Bach-oratory, and the tall trees will appear as mystic gothic cathedrals. Your heart will rejoice, your earthly problems will seem unimportant, and you'll feel happy to be alive. You will count your blessings instead of your problems. And you will be amazed how your mental activity will be sharpened and how thoughts and new ideas will flow with ease.

All in all, your first fasting will be a wonderful experience, which will recharge, renew and rejuvenate your whole personality – body, mind and spirit!

Chapter 10

Dry Brush Massage- A Million Dollar Health and Beauty Secret

How many times have you heard that "the great truths are always simple?" Man has a peculiar fancy for the complicated, involved and elaborate. He has a great respect for things so complex he can't grasp. He is fascinated by the detective work of scientists trying to untangle the "Gordian knot," to solve an inextricable maze.

Indeed, one of the main reasons why, in an age of moon-landings, we are not able to cure or prevent a simple cold, is that scientists are unwilling to recognize the obvious relation between man's ills and his obedience to the simple laws of nature. That such a simple thing as what man eats or doesn't eat could be the cause of most of his ills, is too simple, too unsophisticated a deduction. It is much more glamorous to engage in an elaborate detective hunt in the secret compounds of a complex laboratory, enveloped in an aura of scientific mystery and public adoration, trying to find a viscious germ, or invisi threatens man's health and welfare. For examp fronted with an irrefutable fact that a certain plan by man for thousands of years for the prevention certain disease, the scientist will never be satisfied t endorse or sanction its use – no, he will exhaust all his scie brain power and ingenuity, and, through painstaking research, t to *isolate* the "active ingredient" of the plant, and – hailing a triumphant scientific discovery – present it to a grateful disease-ridden mankind in the form of a white pill!

What I am going to present to you in this chapter would never excite a pill-oriented modern scientist. He would say, "It is too simple to be true", forgetting the great lesson of history that great truths are always simple. For instance, the present-day antibiotics, which scientists "discovered" under such a fanfare, had been used by Indians for centuries in the form of moulded dough or moulded tortillas.

I am going to reveal to you a simple technique, which will cost you a total of fifty cents, which will take only 5 to 10 minutes a day to perform, but which will give you a million dollars worth of benefits in terms of better health, better looks, and longer life. I am deliberately allocating a whole chapter on this secret, so convinced am I of its importance. I have tested it for 25 years on myself and hundred of patients and students. The technique is called *dry brush massage.* It is described in my books, *THERE IS A CURE FOR ARTHRITIS* and *HEALTH SECRETS FROM EUROPE,* and mentioned in chapter 9 of this book. I have received numerous glowing reports of great benefits derived by those who incorporate this simple method into their daily routine.

How do you take dry the brush massage.

First, you have to get a suitable brush. The best brush for massage is a natural-bristle brush about the size of your hand, or larger if you can get it. Unfortunately, it is more and more difficult to find natural bristle brushes, especially in the United States. I buy most of my brushes from Sweden. The brush reach all parts of your body. le brush right away, but are assage program immediately, ry:

al plant-fiber vegetable brush rug store or hardware store. d hogs' hair.

al sponge.

synthetic fiber brushes – they skin.

to start out with a less harsh brush, and brush gently at first, until your skin is "seasoned", then start using a coarser brush.

Starting with the soles of your feet, brush vigorously making rotary motions, and massage every part of your body. Press brush against your body as much as you can comfortably stand. Sensitivity of the skin varies, of course, with every individual. Some can stand much harder brushing than others. Also, the various parts of the body vary in sensitivity. The face, the inner part of the thighs, the abdomen and the chest are the most sensitive parts. Brush in this order: first feet and legs, then hands and arms, the back, abdomen, chest and neck.

Brush until your skin becomes rosy, warm and glowing. Five to ten minutes is the average time, although some people like to brush longer. But do not scrub all your skin off! Everything is best in moderation, including your dry brush massage.

The best time for dry brush massage is upon arising in the morning and again before going to bed.

Massage followed by shower

After dry brush massage it is advisable to take a shower or rub-down with a sponge or wet towel, to wash away dead skin particles. Brushing loosens up copious amounts of dead layers of skin that you can see as a dust on your body.

There are two ways to go about taking a shower. One, used mostly by the patients in European clinics, is the alternating hot and cold shower, followed by dry brush massage. First, take a hot shower for 3 minutes or so, until you feel warmed up, then a cold shower for about 10 to 20 seconds. Repeat this three times, always finishing with cold, as cold as you can stand. After this hot-and-cold shower, rub yourself dry with a coarse towel and then give yourself a brush massage that will warm you up thoroughly.

The other way, which is most suitable for relatively healthy people, is to take the dry brush massage first and finish with alternating hot-and-cold shower, drying and warming up after the shower with a coarse towel. Of course, if you can not tolerate the hot-and-cold shower, you can have a warm shower only. But the alternating hot-and-cold shower has an exceedingly beneficial and stimulating effect on all the vital functions of your body, particularly on the glandular activity. It also stimulates your blood circulation and your nervous system, and has a rejuvenating effect on your skin. The combination of the dry brush massage and a hot-and-cold shower is an excellent way to start and finish your day.

Why dry brush massage is so beneficial

As you have learned before in this book, the number one cause of all so-called degenerative diseases and premature aging is to be found in the derangement of cell metabolism and in slowed-down cell regeneration. This derangement is mainly caused by the accumulation of the waste products in the tissues which interefere with the nourishment and oxygenation of the cells.

Normally, under ideal circumstances, your body cleanses itself automatically without any conscious effort on your part. It is an ingeniously designed self-cleansing, self-protecting and self-healing mechanism. Self-cleansing work is performed by a large group of specially designed organs, glands and transportation systems: alimentary canal, kidneys, liver, lungs, skin, lympathic system, mucous membranes of various cavities, etc. But your largest eliminative organ is the *skin.*

It is estimated that one-third of all body impurities are excreted through the skin. Doctors often refer to the skin as "the third kidney" – and very appropriately so. Hundreds of thousands of tiny sweat glands act not only as the regulators of body temperature, but also as small kidneys, detoxifying organs, ready to cleanse the blood and free the system from health-threatening poisons. The chemical analysis of sweat shows that it has almost the same constituents as urine. Uric acid, the main metabolic waste product, and a normal component of urine, is found in large amount in the perspiration. If the skin becomes inactive and its pores choked with millions of dead cells, uric acid and other impurities will remain in the body. The other eliminative organs, mainly the liver and kidneys, will have to increase their labor of detoxification because of the inactive skin, with the result that they will be overworked and eventually weakened or diseased. Toxins and wastes will then be deposited in the tissues. Thus, you must realize the great importance of keeping your skin always in perfect working condition.

The eliminative capacity of the skin is demonstrated by the fact that more than one pound of waste products is discharged through the skin every day. This explains why man discovered the healing effect of sweating very early in history. The Finnish sauna, and the Turkish, Russian and Roman baths have been used for healing purposes for thousands of years. The famous seventeenth-century Dutch physician, Sylvius, said, "One third of all diseases can be cured by sweating."

In addition to its eliminative work, skin has many other vital functions. The body actually breathes through the skin, absorbing oxygen and exhaling carbon dioxide which is formed in the tissues. Also, through the skin certain nutrients are absorbed into the body. Russian scientific studies show that minerals from the seawater and sea air are absorbed through the skin during seashore holidays. Other scientific studies have demonstrated that skin is capable of assimilating various vitamins, minerals and even proteins applied directly to the skin. It has been long known, too, that by a mysterious chemical process, vitamin D is manufactured on the skin by the influence of the sun rays on the oils produced by the skin glands. Subsequently, vitamin D is absorbed into the system through the skin.

As you can see, your skin is a living, vital organ with a multiplicity of important functions. The tragedy is that the skin of modern man is the most neglected and mistreated organ. In our sheltered, air-conditioned existence skin is seldom exposed to life-giving fresh air or to stimulating temperature changes. How many times this week have you worked or exercised outdoors hard enough to cause profuse perspiration? Dry brush massage will give your skin stimulation, exercise and cleansing of which it is deprived by your sedentary way of life.

Here is an impressive list of benefits you derive from regular dry brush massage:

1. It will effectively remove the dead layers of skin and other impurities and keep pores open.

2. It will stimulate and increase blood circulation in all underlying organs and tissues, and especially in the small blood capillaries of your skin.

3. It will revitalize and increase the eliminative capacity of your skin and help to throw toxins out of the system.

4. It will stimulate the hormone- and oil-producing glands.

5. It has a powerful rejuvenating influence on the nervous system by stimulating nerve endings in the skin.

6. It will help prevent colds, especially when used in combination with hot-and-cold showers.

7. It will contribute to a healthier muscle tone and a better distribution of fat deposits.

8. It will rejuvenate the complexion and make it look younger, fresher and more velvety.

9. It will make you feel better all over and look younger.

10. It will improve your health generally, and help prevent premature aging.

Since the dry brush massage also happens to be one of the most *pleasant* and enjoyable do-it-yourself health measures, don't you think that the above list is impressive enough to convince you to give this million-dollar health and beauty secret an honest try? I am quite confident that once you try it, you will be "sold on it" for the rest of your life!

Some important tips on dry brush massage

1. Every two weeks or so wash your brush with soap and water and dry it in the sun or in a warm place. Your brush will be rapidly filled with impurities and should be washed regularly.
2. For hygenic reasons, use seperate brushes for each member of the family.
3. Avoid brushing the parts of your skin that are irritated, damaged or infected.
4. The scalp should be brushed, too. For scalp brushing a good bristle brush is a must – no other substitute will do. Scalp brushing will stimulate hair growth by increasing blood circulation, and keep scalp clean from dandruff, stale oils and other impurities.
5. The facial skin of most people is too sensitive for brushing, so it is better to leave it alone.
6. If you don't have a brush with an extended handle, ask your husband or wife to help you with the brushing. Brush massage is doubly enjoyable when somebody else gives it to you. Mutual morning and evening brush massage session may even add a new dimension to your marriage!
7. An excellent way to improve the quality of your skin and the looks of your complexion is to rub or massage your whole body with a nourishing oil immediately after dry brushing. Any cold-pressed vegetable oil, obtainable at health food stores, can be used. I particularly recommend the following oils: sesame oil, avocado oil, almond oil. Or, still better, use my FORMULA F. You can make this natural cosmetic in your own kitchen.

FORMULA F

5 tbsp. sesame oil
3 tbsp. olive oil

4 tbsp. a
2 tbsp. a
1 tbsp.
A few

All the above oils can be
Pour all the ingredients in
tightly and shake well. Keep in refrigerator.

Formula F is composed of the most beautifying oils known
man and it will do wonders for your skin. Do not use too much; a few drops of the formula will go far. Apply more on the face, neck, hand and arms. It will make your skin look moist, soft, and velvety beautiful. It will also help to prevent wrinkles and premature aging of the skin.

Chapter 11

The Water Controversies

There is no longer controversy in regard to our polluted waters. Only a decade ago or so those of us who talked about the slow mass suicide that we were committing by polluting the waters in lakes and rivers were called alarmists. But now, everyone is suddenly aware of the grave consequences we have to face for abusing our water supplies. The President of the United States told us, in his 1970 State of the Union speech, that we have to clean our environment or perish. I am afraid that it might be "perish", because, in spite of all the talk and promises, nothing is being or will be done; more toxic matter than ever before is pouring into our lakes and rivers from industrial sources, from fields and forests saturated with chemical fertilizers and toxic sprays, and from sewage loaded with household detergents and other poisonous chemicals. We may have already reached the point of no return.

Since there is general agreement now on the subject of polluted water, and since this book deals with controversies, misconceptions and confusion, we will discuss a few other controversial topics regarding water.

Fluoridation of the water

Let me state clearly and loudly that fluoridation of the water is the *biggest hoax in medical history perpetrated on innocent people in the name of science.*

Some 80 million Americans are now mass-medicated by toxic sodium fluoride, while there is *no positive, conclusive, scientific proof* that the addition of this inorganic toxic chemical does the least bit of good, even to the teeth of children between ages 7 and 12. But there are dozens of reliable studies made around the world that show that the fluoridation of the water causes fluorosis (mottling of tooth enamel), mongolism in infants, kidney damage, and other harmful effects to the body by its direct effect, and by its interference with enzyme, mineral and vitamin functions within the system. These studies are, however, suppressed; researchers are persecuted; and their findings are not published in medical journals. Woe to those who dare to go against the orthodoxy's monopoly of thoughts, ideas and practices!

Unfortunately, space limitations prevent us from going into detail about this fascinating question of misguided chemical "progress", fluoridation of the water. Suffice here to say that several governments in Europe – notably Denmark, Poland, Sweden, Russia and Italy – have investigated all American claims for the benefits and safety of fluoridation and, after careful study, have *prohibited fluoridation by law* – on the grounds that "there is not sufficient evidence as to the benefit or the safety of this unscientific measure". The Swedish government and the Swedish Medical Society have for several years campaigned *for* water fluoridation, but in 1970 reversed their policy, and now are advising to stop all future fluoridation. A committee of forty Swedish medical experts, after a careful study of the newest facts, reported that "because of the increasing amount of reports which link artificially fluoridated water to a variety of health-damaging effects, all further fluoridation of the water in Sweden should be stopped until more knowledge of harmful side-effects of water fluoridation is obtained."

(Those who are interested in studying the fluoridation question thoroughly should read the most informative book on the subject, called FLUORIDATION, compiled by the National Health Federation and obtainable from *NHF, P.O. Box 686, Monrovia, California, 91016.)*

Just one more thought on fluoridation – not a very scientific, but a *plain horse-sense thought.* The American Dental Association supports and endorses fluoridation very forcefully and spends a lot of its members' money on pro-fluoridation campaigns, advertising and propaganda, pushing fluoridation down the throats of the American people. Pro-fluoridationist doctors and dentists claim that mass-fluoridation would reduce the tooth decay by 60 per cent. Are you naïve enough to believe that the American dentists, in mass, would endorse and *actually financially support a program that would reduce their income by 60 per cent?* They are not that dumb. They know that fluoridation of water will not reduce their incomes. *There are actually as many or more dentists in the towns with 15 or more years of fluoridation than there are in non-fluoridated towns of comparable size.* Fluoridation results in mottled teeth which need lots of dental work later in life and early replacement by dentures. You may not know what *you* are doing when you vote for the fluoridation of your water supply, but pro-fluoridationists know what *they* are doing – believe me! If they are so genuinely interested in reducing tooth decay – and reducing their incomes – by 60%, why don't they try advocating sugar-free diets and bone-meal supplements? It has been demonstrated conclusively by several researchers in Sweden and in the United States that such simple prophylactics as the addition of bone-meal to the diet and the avoidance of white sugar and white bread will bring tooth decay to a virtual standstill. In a Swedish study, children brought up on bone-meal supplements were almost 100 per cent free from tooth decay. Why don't the American dentists push this kind of caries-preventive program, *which really works?*

Abraham Lincoln said: "You can fool some of the people all of the time, and all of the people some of the time, but you can not fool all of the people all of the time." Almost one half of the American people have now been fooled for 20 years. Will *all* of the American people have to be fooled for "some of the time," before they will finally be awakened to the fact that they have been used as the guinea pigs of a quasi-scientific experiment based on an erroneous, speculative theory?

Distilled vis-à-vis natural water

There has been a great deal of confusion lately in regard to the advisability of drinking distilled water. Some health "experts" tell us that all well water, spring water, lake water, and fresh, running river and stream water is not good for human consumption. We know that practically all fresh water is polluted these days; and all the health experts agree that we *should* drink only pure, fresh, unpolluted and uncontaminated water that hasn't been chlorinated or fluoridated. These are not the points of disagreement in this controversy, however. The reason some experts condemn all natural water is that "it contains large amounts of inorganic minerals which the body can not use." The same experts claim that these inorganic minerals can cause stiff joints, hardening of the arteries, gallstones, kidney and bladder stones, and many other ills. They advise, therefore, that the only "natural" water which is good for you is steam-processed distilled water.

This distilled water idea is one of the most nonsensical and unscientific fads that has hit the health business in a long while.

Consider these *facts:*

1. Man has used natural waters from springs, rivers and lakes for thousands of years, and enjoyed wonderful health. Hardening of the arteries is a relatively recent disease, a disease of civilization.
2. *All* wild animals drink natural waters and enjoy perfect health and complete freedom from disease.
3. The Hunza people, known for their extraordinary health and *total freedom from hardening of the arteries or gallbladder or kidney stones,* drink natural waters that contain even more inorganic minerals than the waters in other parts of the world.

4. It has been scientifically established that in many places of the world, notably one town in England, where drinking water is extremely "hard", i. e. it contains extra large amounts of minerals, the people have a much lower incidence of arteriosclerosis as compared to the areas where people drink so-called "soft" water.
5. The latest findings of the British Society for the Advancement of Science and the U.S. Navy Dental Research Institute show that drinking so-called hard water, which is rich in minerals and trace elements, particularly molybdenum, strontium and flourine, can prevent tooth decay and cardio-vascular diseases, caused by the hardening of the arteries. The trace element chromium in hard water helps to prevent diabetes.
6. Distilled water, void of all minerals, is *not* a *natural* water. It is a synthetic, artificial, man-made, fragmented product that does not occur "naturally". Prolonged drinking of soft (read: deficient in minerals) or distilled water will result in mineral deficiences and lead to deficiency-caused diseases.

There is no scientific evidence whatsoever that minerals from the water plug the arteries and cause arteriosclerosis. Hardening of the arteries is caused by the cholesterol deposits on the inside walls of the blood vessels. Some calcium and other minerals may be deposited on cholesterol, but this is not caused by drinking hard water, but by faulty mineral metabolism.

Organic versus inorganic minerals

The main objection against drinking natural waters is that they contain inorganic minerals that the body "can not use". This objection is based on the antiquated theory that our body can use only the organic minerals. All minerals, chemicals, metals, salts and trace elements that are present in plant and animal tissues are *organic*. Those minerals that are present in soil, rocks, water, sea water, and air are *inorganic*. As plants grow, they transform inorganic minerals into organic minerals.

It may be true that your body can *use* only organic minerals, if with the word *use* we mean the body's ability to assimilate and utilize these minerals as essential building blocks for renewal and repair of cells, and for many other vital biochemical and metabolic processes in the system.

This does not mean, however, that inorganic minerals can not be absorbed into the system, that they are completely useless. There is some recent research which suggests that inorganic minerals, which have always been an integral part of man's environment, have some important part to play in man's life processes.

For example, people have been using mineral springs and various kinds of mineral water baths for ages, long before civilization. I have seen ancient bathing places in the Caucassus mountains of Russia, where cave dwellers carried their sick to bathe in natural hot mineral springs. I have seen many such ancient bathing places, balnearios, in Mexico. Mexican Indians have been using mineral waters for the healing of their sick since long before any white man stepped on this continent. They also use mineral-rich seawater to cure themselves of diseases. I have met many Indian medicine men who employ seawater and sand packs, and who recommend drinking seawater for many ailments. In Germany, I have visited dozens of mineral water Spas, where millions of people take "cures".

Note that all these mineral waters, as well as seawater, contain only *inorganic minerals.* If your body can not use them at all, if they do nothing but cause serious disorders and diseases, as you have been told, then why do millions of people around the world visit these Spas and mineral springs and report enthusiastically of the many health benefits, even cures, they obtain from them?

The medicinal value of mineral water

The medicinal and health-promoting properties of mineral waters have been demonstrated in many experiments and studies.

Drs. Korenyi, Harkavy and Whittier reported on the experiments they conducted with 34 patients with high cholesterol levels at the Greedmoor State Hospital in New York. These patients, whose serum cholesterol levels were above 240 mg.%, did not receive any other type treatment known to have any effect on serum cholesterol, except 30.5 fluid ounces of mineral water daily in three divided doses. The treatment continued 30 days.

At the end of two weeks the average decrease of serum cholesterol was 9.9 mg.%. At the conclusion of the study, the average decrease was 23.8mg.%.

A Hungarian doctor, O. Schulhof, M.D., made a study of mineral Spa therapies and reported that "beside the psychological effects produced by the changed environment, and the complex effect of other therapeutic treatments, we still attribute importance to the specific effect of the mineral water." Dr. Schulhof said that it has been demonstrated that mineral water is actually absorbed through the skin. According to Dr. Schulhof, mineral waters have a beneficial effect on the connective tissues as well as on the immunological and healing powers of the body.

In Germany, three million people frequent mineral bathing and drinking Spas each year, most of them on their doctors' recommendations. In Bad Pyrmont, I visited the famous Mineral Water Cure establishment run and directed by the State Medical Board. Medical doctors supervise the "water cures" at Bad Pyrmont. Here is a quote from the brochure published by the State Medical Government:

"Bad Pyrmont Spa facilities are recommended for the treatment of the following diseases: diseases of the heart and circulation; cardiac insufficiency, cardiac infarct, coronary thrombosis; disorders in blood pressure, peripheral circulation disorders; nervous disorders, diseases of the blood-forming organs; all types of anemia; rheumatic diseases of the bones, joints and muscles; women's complaints: inflammation of female abdominal organs, periodic and other hormone disorders; eczema; allergies; conditions of exhaustion; children's diseases; diseases of old age and senility."

Keep in mind that this is not a "quack"-operated joint trying to cheat people of their money, offering bogus mineral water cures for all these serious diseases, but a *State-operated Spa that has been approved by the State Medical Association!*

If mineral waters didn't work or did not have a beneficial and curative effect, do you think these hundreds of mineral Spas would be operated on such a grand scale for thousands of years?

A doctor with whom I spoke at Bad Pyrmont told me: "The modern inquiry into Balnealogy* and the medicinal value of mineral waters is recent and as yet incomplete. But what is already known indicates that mineral waters do indeed have a curative effect. And they should, inasmuch as disorders in mineral metabolism and biochemical derangement are at the root of many diseases. But what is even more important is the fact that these mineral waters have been used for healing purposes for almost two thousands years; and millions of sick people have been benefitted by them – patients and doctors see examples of it every day."

In our own experience directing biological therapies at a mineral water Spa in Mexico, many of our patients have recovered quite spectacularly on a combined biological program of fasting, special diets and hot mineral baths. We also advised them to drink one glass of mineral water each day. Patients with high blood pressure, arthritis, vericose veins, thyroid insufficiency, asthma, psoriasis, and cardiac and circulatory disorders have responded rather miraculously to the Spa therapy. Many arthritics who were badly incapacitated and immobile, have walked for miles in hilly terrain after a few weeks of treatment; patients with high blood pressure improved dramatically, showing decreases in blood pressure of 30 to 40 mm. after 2 weeks; and patients with respiratory and heart problems experienced great relief within a few weeks.

The available research work, corroborated by our own experience, suggests that inorganic minerals present in seawater and mineral waters have a definite curative effect on many disorders by *stimulating the body's own defensive and healing forces.*

---

*Balnealogy – the Medical Science of curing and preventing sickness by bathing.

My assumption is that the healing effect of mineral water is not only due to the nutritive value of the minerals present, but also to the catalytic effect of these minerals on the vital biochemical body processes.

The health-building value of minerals in water scientifically confirmed.

Recently, the British Society for the Advancement of Science held a special Congress in Exeter, England, to study the effects of minerals and trace elements in man's environment – water, air and soil – on man's health. It was revealed at the Congress, as an established fact, that in the areas where people drink water rich in trace elements molybdenum, strontium and fluorine, they have less caries, or tooth decay. It has been also established that in the areas where drinking water is deficient in trace element chromium, there is an abnormally high prevalence of diabetes. The Congress has specifically stressed the fact, based on latest findings, that the so-called hard water (water with high mineral content) has a definite preventive effect against the development of cardio-vascular diseases caused by arteriosclerosis, or hardening of the arteries. The fact was considered "remarkable" because hard water contains more calcium than soft water.

A very convincing discovery, proving the value of drinking so-called hard water (rich in minerals and trace elements), was made by Drs. Losee and Adkins at U.S. Navy Dental Research Institute. Checking in the birthplaces and homes of 360 recruits who never had a single dental cavity in their lives, the researchers discovered the remarkable fact that they all lived in three small geographic regions of the United States – northwest Ohio, northeast South Carolina and west central Florida. Set out to discover what circumstances peculiar to these areas caused people to resist dental decay, the scientists discovered that the water supplies in these areas were rich in minerals and trace elements, particularly in molybdenum and strontium, but also boron and lithium. Hard, mineralized water the cavity-free recruits were drinking all their lives, was "significantly higher" in these minerals than the water in the other areas of the country known for the average amount of dental cavities. For example, there was 50 times as much strontium in the water samples from northwest Ohio as in the water from the high-cavity states.

The researchers, impressed by the cavity-resistant property of minerals and trace elements in drinking water, conducted controlled experiments with rats to prove their discovery scientifically. Four groups of rats were given special dental decay-producing diets plus distilled water (devoid of minerals), fluoridated water, artifically mineralized water and natural mineral-rich water. The group that drank natural water containing minerals and trace elements was "significantly better" both in numbers and severity of dental decay. Incidentally, the group that drank fluoridated water, showed no improvement in dental health over the groups which drank unfluoridated water.

Since dental health is a very reliable indication of overall health, the above research clearly demonstrates the wisdom and health-building value of drinking hard, naturally mineralized water rich in tooth-health minerals, particularly in molybdenum and strontium.

Dr. Ragnar Berg, perhaps the world's greatest authority on nutrition and biochemistry, said, "It is extremely important for man's growth and his health that he uses "hard" water for drinking . . . Drinking mineral-rich hard water could improve the calcium-deficient diets of civilized men."

What about seawater?

We have all experienced the invigorating effect of a few days or weeks by the seashore. The reason is this: minerals from the seawater and air are actually absorbed through the skin and lungs.

Health food stores have recently begun selling seawater as a food supplement. Dr. M. O. Garten tells in his book, THE HEALTH SECRETS OF NATUROPATHIC DOCTOR, of many remarkable cases where health was restored to patients given about one ounce of seawater daily. Cases of Parkinson's disease, chronic indigestion, bleeding gums, and other chronic ailments responded dramatically to seawater therapy.

What is the secret of the therapeutic property of seawater? It is an extremely rich source of all the basic minerals of which your body is made. The chemical composition of seawater is about the same as the chemical composition of your blood. But many doctors and researchers seriously doubt that the mere presence of minerals in seawater is responsible for its startling healing property. By drinking only an ounce of seawater a day, patients get such infinitesimal amounts of minerals that their nutritive value, could not possibly be entirely responsible for the good results. I am inclined to believe that, whatever other mysterious forces or principles are invovled in the beneficial effects of seawater, the healing and health-promoting property of seawater is basically due to the catalytic action of the inorganic minerals it contains. The mineral components and the heavy metal salts of seawater act as catalysts to restore disturbed body chemistry, and stimulate the assimilation of organic minerals from foods. The minerals in seawater, which are inorganic, act within the body as chemical stimulants for the body s various organs and glands, regenerating and normalizing the functions of these organs and stimulating and increasing the body's own healing forces. The homeopathic doses of minerals from ionized seawater, with its life-giving chemo-electrical and cosmic forces, are quickly absorbed into the system where they have a healing effect on all body cells, nerve tissues, glands and vital organs.

Summary

In view of all the evidence, both scientific and empirical, of the beneficial therapeutic and prophylactic effect of mineral waters, seawater and plain natural "living" drinking water from springs, rivers or lakes – which all contain inorganic minerals – how can anyone claim that these waters are harmful and that you should drink only steam-processed distilled water? To call the man-made, processed, artificially distilled water "natural" is to pervert the meaning of the word. "Natural" is something you can find in nature as an integral part of the God-made universe. Of all the natural waters upon this earth none is distilled. Rainwater is naturally distilled, but become mineralized when it reaches rivers and lakes. There are a few small tribes living in desert areas who are forced to collect rainwater for drinking; but they do so only because of necessity. When natural lake or stream water is available, man always choses it for drinking and cooking. There is no evidence that the rainwater-drinking tribes enjoy better health. But there is plenty of evidence showing that people who drink the natural, mineralized waters of mountain streams, springs and lakes have always enjoyed superior health. To "prove" the superiority of distilled water by telling how great a single individual feels who has been drinking it for decades, is no more scientific than to use cigar-smoking and whiskey-drinking Churchill, who lived to be 92, as proof of the health-giving properties of cigars and whiskey.

Those who drink distilled water and feel good, do so not because of the distilled water but *in spite of it.* Switch back to natural, mineral-rich, sun-drenched, oxygenized and ionized "living" water from flowing springs and streams, and take some mineral water or small amounts of seawater occasionally – and feel the difference this change will make!

Unfortunately, it is becoming more and more difficult to obtain natural "living" water from flowing springs and streams in the United States. Practically all inland sweet water is contaminated by sewage, pesticides, detergents, etc. To city tap water has been added many more toxic chemicals to the previously contaminated water – such as chlorine, fluorine, and many more. So the only way to assure pure water supply in the United States today is to buy bottled water which is on sale in most supermarkets. Both natural, pure spring water, as well as distilled water, are available. I trust that after reading this chapter you will make the right choice when you buy your bottled water.

Chapter 12

Vitamin P– The Controversial Healer

Most people are familiar with vitamins A, B, C, D, and E. A few have heard of the less known vitamins H, F, K, and U. But what about vitamin P? The American Medical Association and FDA have persistently and determinately ignored vitamin P – known in the United States generally as the bioflavonoids – which *European research has demonstrated to be among the most important nutritive substances.* AMA's Council on Drugs claims that bioflavonoids are "of little or no value" in the treatment of disease. And very recently, FDA has taken a direct action to withdraw bioflavonoids from the American market on the basis that they are ineffective and worthless.

Bioflavonoids – what they are

Bioflavonoids are natural substances which occur in fruits and vegetables, particularly in those containing vitamin C. They were discovered by Hungarian physician and Nobel Prize Winner,

Dr. Albert Szent-Gyorgyi, in 1936. Dr. Szent-Gyorgyi isolated vitamin C from oranges in 1927. At the time it was presumed that the vitamin C was the sole active substance in citrus fruits which were known to benefit patients with bleeding problems. It was soon found, however, that vitamin C in its pure form (ascorbic acid) was not sufficiently effective when given alone in certain types of bleeding. In 1936, Dr. Szent-Gyorgyi succeeded in isolating a group of substances from lemons and green peppers which were found to be effective in cases that did not respond to treatment with vitamin C alone. These substances were found to have a curative action on the permeability of capillaries, and therefore were called Vitamin P.

Vitamin P, or bioflavonoids, are always combined with vitamin C in nature; in fact they seem to be a part of the vitamin C complex. Some of the identified bioflavonoids are rutin, hesperidin and citrin. Medically known as *flavone glycosides,* they are found mostly in green peppers, buckwheat, citrus fruits, grapes, rose hips, apricots, black currants, acerola cherries, and many other fruits and vegetables where also vitamin C is naturally present.

During the past 30 years many research projects and clinical investigations have been undertaken on the prophylactic and therapeutic properties of the bioflavonoids. Over 500 scientific papers on bioflavonoids have been published in reputable medical journals around the world. In 1959, a scientific symposium on bioflavonoids was held in Moscow, entitled *Vitamin P – Its Properties and Its Uses.* It was revealed at the symposium that Russians have used bioflavonoids very successfully in treatment of many diseases, particularly in capillary fragility. The clinical reports from around the world have shown that vitamin P therapy is effective in such diversified conditions as rheumatic fever, spontaneous abortions or miscarriages, high blood pressure, respiratory infections, hemorrhaging, bleeding gums, eczema, psoriasis, hemorrhoids, cirrhosis of the liver, etc. Vitamin P is also useful as a protective agent against the harmful effects of X-rays.

Why vitamin P is ignored in the U. S.

Why then should the FDA ignore and deny the importance of Vitamin P in nutrition, and in therapeutic medicine, and even go as far as to try to ban the sale of bioflavonoids in the United States? Vitamin P, like vitamin C, is completely harmless and has no toxicity whatever, even in massive doses. While there are thousands of potentially harmful, toxic and dangerous drugs on the market, which could and should be investigated, why is the FDA trying to ban totally harmless vitamin P and make it unavailable to the American public? Has the fact that bioflavonoids are *natural substances* that can not be produced synthetically anything to do with it? Perhaps bioflavonoids are associated with food faddism in the minds of the FDA directors, since health food stores and health publications were first to promote bioflavonoids and bring them to the attention of the public.

Whatever the answer, the failure of American medicine to accept and use vitamin P as a valid therapeutic agent is a definite detriment to the health of the American people. Ascorbic acid, the pure synthetic form of vitamin C, is used now widely in the United States. But vitamin C is much more potent when it is combined with bioflavonoids. They are *synergists* – i.e. the combined effect of these two substances administered together is greater than the sum of the individual effects. Much of the clinical and laboratory research was incomplete and misleading because this *synergistic effect of vitamins C and P was not taken into consideration.*

Here are some of the scientific experiments and research done by European scientists with vitamin P.

Hemorrhoids

Dr. Bernard A. D. Wissmer of the Medical Polyclinic of the University of Geneva has cured thousands of patients suffering from various types of hemorrhoids with a bioflavonoid trioxyethylrutin, referred to as vitamin P_4. In most cases, pain and hemorrhage ceased after 2 to 5 days of treatment. No adverse side effects were noticed although several thousand patients received the treatment.

Another Swiss physician, Dr. Igor Berson, has reported that the results in a series of treatments on hemorrhoids with bioflavonoids were "extremely encouraging". Report says that due to the decongestive action of vitamin P_4, pain, pruritus (itch), and often even hemorrhoids "disappeared entirely".

Respiratory infections

Drs. W. C. Martin and M. S. Biskind, of Australia, in their famous study on 22 cases of cold, influenza and tonsillitis treated with vitamin P, observed a dramatic remission of symptoms in 20 cases. In many cases, recovery occurred as soon as 8 hours after beginning of the treatment. The report says that bioflavonoids were effective no matter in what stage of infection the treatment was started.

Russian experiments with mice infected with influenza virus showed that while only 9.4 per cent of untreated animals survived, in the group treated with vitamin P, 31.9 per cent survived the infection.

High blood pressure

In the Russian report on *Vitamin P and its Properties,* Dr. G. S. Koroza tells of long-term animal experiments on treatment of hypertension with vitamin P. He used 50 mg. of vitamin P per kilogram of body weight. A 15-20 mm. of mercury fall in blood pressure was noted.

In another study, Dr. D. E. Dzheims-Levi has reported that the blood pressure of patients with hypertension was "considerably lowered" after the administration of vitamin P. It was also noted that when the patients discontinued vitamin P treatment blood pressure rose again.

Varicose veins

Dr. Igor Berson, consulting phlebologist of the Dermatological Clinic of the University of Lausanne, Switzerland, reported that of 1,396 patients with varicose veins, hemorrhoids, chronic venous insufficiency, and inflammation of the capillaries, 1,100 showed fair to good results after therapy with vitamin P_4. The use of P_4 was hailed as the first important progress in the treatment of varicose veins and other venous diseases.

Other conditions

There is much corroborative research done in the United States and other countries on the use of vitamin P in a variety of conditions. It has been demonstrated that vitamin P protects against the effects of radiation; mortality rate of rats exposed to X-rays was reduced 800 per cent by the use of the vitamin. Gum bleeding was stopped by the administration of bioflavonoids and vitamin C. Vitamin P was also shown to be successful in the treatment of habitual abortions, rheumatic fever and anemia.

How vitamin P works

The main property of vitamin P is its ability to increase the strength of the capillaries and regulate their permeability. There are millions of miles of tiny blood vessels, capillaries, which connect the arteries and veins in the tissues. Vitamin P is also known to assist vitamin C in keeping collagen, the intercellular cement, in a healthy condition. These properties of vitamin P help to prevent hemorrhages and ruptures in capillaries and connective tissues, speed the healing of wounds, and build a protective barrier against infections. It is generally known that the majority of viral and bacterial infections, as well as many of the chronic degenerative diseases, such as arthritis and cardiovascular disorders, are accompanied by disturbances in capillary permeability and loss of strength and stability in capillaries and the collagen. The Russian Symposium on Vitamin P stated that capillary disturbances are often found in such diseases as lung tuberculosis, rheumatic fever, high blood pressure, diabetes, poliomyelitis, smallpox and measles.

It can be readily seen, therefore, why vitamin P, with its amazing power of capillary-strengthening action, is such an effective agent in the prevention and correction of so many different disorders.

Application

HOW TO USE VITAMIN P FOR PREVENTION AND TREATMENT OF DISEASE

If you suffer from any of the conditions named in this chapter and have tried conventional treatments without success, you may want to try vitamin P. The studies reported here have all been conducted by reputable scientists under scientific controls. If you have an unprejudiced doctor, ask him if vitamin P treatment would be advisable in your case. Of course, bioflavonoids are completely harmless, so there is no danger in using them as supplements, just like any other vitamins. Don't forget the *synergistic action* of vitamins P and C – *take them always together for the greater effect.* The usual doses used in reported studies were from 100 to 200 mg. capsules. Children can safely take 100 mg. three times a day; adults 4-6 times or more. But even 1,000 to 2,000 mg. per day would be perfectly safe.

HOW TO PLAN A DIET RICH IN VITAMIN P

For preventive purposes, for building up the capillary strength and adequate resistance to infections, see that your diet contains plenty of raw fruits and vegetables rich in bioflavonoids. Citrus fruits, green peppers, grapes, apricots, strawberries, and black currants are especially rich in vitamin P. Most of the other berries and fruits are also good sources; but they must be eaten fresh and raw. Bioflavonoids are largely destroyed by cooking and preserving.

Note: a glass of orange juice in the morning does not guarantee that you get your supply of bioflavonoids. They are mostly in the white pulp of the fruits and in the sheaths separating the sections in citrus. So when you squeeze your juice you leave most of the bioflavonoids in the orange peels. Don't drink your fruits – eat them! This applies to citrus fruits perhaps even more so than to other fruits. The citric acid in citrus juices can have a detrimental effect on teeth and on the digestive tract, if consumed in excess.

One of the best and the safest ways to assure plenty of bioflavonoids in your diet is to supplement it with rose hips. There must be a reason why these "vitamin roses" grow so abundantly in the cold northern sections of the globe. Rose hips contain up to 30 times more vitamin C than oranges and are extremely rich in bioflavonoids. The people of northern Europe – Norwegians, Swedes, Finns, and Russians – eat plenty of rose hips and fortify themselves against the cold rugged climate in which they live. Rose hips are available in the United States from health food stores in a whole, powder, or tablet form. They can be used as a tea, sprinkled over cereals or other foods or taken as a food supplement.

Whatever way you take your vitamin P, see that you get ample amounts of it. *The prophylactic and therapeutic properties of vitamin P are too vast to be ignored.*

Chapter 13

What Can You Do About Hair Loss and Baldness?

The problem of hair loss, or baldness, is as old as man himself. Through the ages men have desperately tried countless methods to stop hair loss and grow more hair – unsuccessfully. Many theories existed as to the cause of baldness, but none of them was proven to be scientifically valid. Circulation problems, pressure by hats, nutritional deficiencies, mental stress of heavy intellectual work – all these and many more theories can be dismissed by one question – why men only? Certainly, women are subjected to the same mental stress, blood circulation problems and nutritional deficiencies. Why is it, then, that women don't get bald, but men do? The pressure on blood capillaries by men's hats was suggested as a possible cause. But now we have a whole generation of men who have grown up without ever having a hat on their heads – yet, baldness is more widespread than ever. Conversely, in countries in Central America and the Far and Middle East, where almost all men wear hats all the time, baldness is virtually unknown.

Is there an answer to the baldness and hair loss problem? Or must the millions of men – and the growing number of women – resign themselves to the inevitable "Nothing can be done"?

Five years ago I wrote a booklet called *STOP HAIR LOSS.* The book brought hopeful news to millions of bald and balding men around the world. It presented to the world the revolutionary Swedish discovery by Dr. Lars Engstrand, M.D., assistant professor at the world-famous Karolinska Medical Institute and Research Center in Stockholm. Dr. Engstrand was the first man who was able to point out *the exact cause of baldness* and prove by his own experiments the correctness of his conclusions.

Dr. Engstrand's method

Working on the problems of pathological conditions in the blood vessel system particularly in the blood circulation of the small capillaries, Dr. Engstrand observed that blood circulation in the scalp was impaired in men more than in women. He discovered that the crown of the head, in both men and women, is covered with a thin sheet-like membrane called the *galea.* It covers the area of the scalp where the typical male-pattern baldness develops. In women, the galea remains thin and elastic throughout life. But in men, approximately from the age of sexual maturity, or 16 to 18 years of age, the galea, through the influence of male sex hormones, gradually becomes thicker and creates a tension and pressure on the blood vessels in the scalp. This pressure hinders the flow of blood to the small blood capillaries which feed the hair follicles with the nutrients necessary for hair growth. The result: a gradual diminishing of hair growth and eventual baldness.

Dr. Engstrand had developed a simple surgical method by which he relieves the pressure in the scalp. He performed thousands of such operations with quite remarkable results. In the most favorable group of patients, between 70 and 80 per cent had experienced increased hair growth within 6 months. Even within completely bald areas his method grew new hair in 40 to 50 per cent of the patients, provided that baldness was of less than 5 years duration.

Dr. Engstrand's research has definitely established that loss of hair and baldness is indeed caused by impaired blood circulation due to effect by the male sex hormones. Men with generous sex hormone production have a greater chance of losing their hair. Dr. Engstrand also stressed that mental and emotional stresses cause tensions in the muscle tissues of the scalp and can contribute to hair loss by constricting the blood vessels.

After my book, *STOP HAIR LOSS,* was published, I received many letters. Among them were a couple from researchers who suggested that Dr. Engstrand's theory that baldness is caused by an enlarged galea and insufficient blood circulation had been disproved by the recent, successful method of hair transplants. If the hair on bald heads fell out because of insufficient blood supply to the scalp, the new hair transplants wouldn't grow on such heads. It had been demonstrated, however, that the newly-transplanted hair thrived and grew vigorously. Faced with such strong counter-evidence, I was ready to discard my belief in Dr. Engstrand's theory and rewrite my book. But then reports began to come in that the hair transplant method turned out to be something less than a great success, in spite of its triumphant introduction. In some patients, transplanted hairs thrived for a while, even as long as a year or more, then gradually their growth began to slow down and eventually hairs fell out. Also, don't forget that during hair transplantation the galea is penetrated and, thus, the pressure on the blood vessels feeding hair roots, eliminated. Dr. Engstrand's concept of baldness was accurate after all.

Can baldness problem be solved by improved nutrition?

Whether or not Dr. Engstrand's surgical approach to increasing the blood supply to the hair roots is the right answer to the problem of hair loss remains to be seen. There are, however, other ways to stimulate increased blood flow to the hair roots. Improved nutrition, with special vitamin supplementation, is one of the successful ways.

The true macrobiotic diet, as outlined in Chapter 3 of this book, is essential for good hair growth. Good general health is imperative for the healthy condition of the scalp. In particular, the digestive system must be working effectively so that the nutrients from the foods you eat will be properly assimilated.

Do not make the mistake of eating *lots of proteins* to prevent hair loss or improve your hair growth. In Chapter 2 of this book I demonstrated that high-animal-protein diet is detrimental to health. What is detrimental to your general health is detrimental to your hair health. Don't be fooled by the reasoning that your hair is made mostly of proteins. Of course, it is made mostly of proteins, so is the rest of your body. This does not mean, however, that you must eat huge amounts of protein each day. All the proteins your hair needs for its daily growth you will probably obtain in one potato or two swallows of milk. Your total protein intake should not exceed 50 to 60 grams per day – which is less than half what is usually advocated in the United States. Proteins eaten in excess of the actual need, especially the animal proteins, are definitely detrimental to your health, including the health of your hair. Did you ever ponder the fact that you rarely see a bald man in Japan, China, India or Mexico? These people have beautiful black hair, and lots of it, as long as they live. *Yet, they live on a very low protein diet, by American standards.*

If you like to undertake a program of feeding your hair from within by improved nutrition, then follow the optimum diet for optimum health – also, for optimum hair health – as outlined in Chapter 3.

"Protein powder" for hair growth

To what extent the Americans are conditioned to think "protein" by the continuous high-protein propaganda is illustrated by the fact that one company has formulated a finely ground powder from well-known "wonder foods" which is sold as a "protein powder". The formula is used mostly as a nutritional help for hair growth. It contains wheat germ, rice polishings, kelp, sunflower seeds, fenugreek, chia seeds and brewer's yeast. All these ingredients are gold-mines of minerals, such as iron, copper, zinc, silicon, phosphorus, calcium, and potassium; vitamins, especially all B-complex vitamins, and vitamins E and A; and natural unsaturated fatty acid – all the ingredients known to be extremely beneficial for better hair growth and prevention of baldness. The formula, of course, also contains a good amount of vegetable proteins. But to call this natural food product, which is extremely rich in hair-growth-promoting minerals, vitamins, trace elements and natural oils, a "protein powder" is to capitalize on the current American high-protein craze. This formula of natural seeds, kelp, yeast, and wheat germ – all known health-builders – is bound to improve the general health of those who use it, including their hair health. But it will work mainly because of it's minerals, B and E vitamins and unsaturated fatty acids it contains, not because of its proteins.

Vitamins and minerals for hair growth

The best way to find out what nutritive substances have a beneficial effect on hair growth is to study the nutritional habits of people who have beautiful hair and don't know what baldness or graying of hair is. As a rule the diet of such people is low in animal proteins (even relatively low in vegetable proteins) but extremely rich in certain vitamins, minerals and essential fatty acids. The diets of these people are rich in whole grains and beans (vitamin B, E, lecithin and unsaturated fatty acids), fresh vegetables and fruits (vitamin C and bioflavonoids.)

Vitamins from the B-complex group which have been demonstrated to be extremely important for your hair are: inositol, choline, biotin, pantothenic acid, PABA, niacin and folic acid.

Vitamin E has been shown to have hair-growth-promoting properties. Vitamin E taken internally oxygenates the blood and stimulates the blood circulation. Used externally (applied to the skin), it increases the blood flow to the skin surface, causing a rise in skin temperature and an increase in blood volume.

Vitamin C is extremely important for the health of the capillaries and all connective tissues.

Vitamin F, or unsaturated fatty acids, is important for the healthy condition of the sebaceous glands. And health of your hair is closely related to the condition of the sebaceous glands.

All minerals are important for the health of the hair, but particularly iodine, copper, iron, silicon, calcium, magnesium, potassium and phosphorus. Vitamin D is important for the proper assimilation of minerals.

Lecithin is very rich in choline, inositol and phosphorus – all acknowledged hair-growth stimulants.

DO-IT-YOURSELF PROGRAM FOR BETTER HAIR GROWTH

Here is a 7-point do-it-yourself program to increase the blood flow to your scalp, stimulate hair growth, and prevent hair loss and baldness – and possibly even grow new hair on already bald heads.

1. Eat the optimum macrobiotic diet of vital foods, as described in Chapter 3 of this book. Emphasis should be on the whole grains, seeds and nuts, eaten predominantly raw or sprouted. Sunflower seeds, sesame seeds, chia seeds, and all nuts are especially beneficial.
2. Supplement your diet with the following B-vitamin-packed foods:
   - Brewer's yeast, powder or flakes – 2 to 3 tablespoons a day.
   - Lecithin, granules – 1 to 2 tablespoons a day.
   - Raw wheat germ – 2 to 3 tablespoons a day.
3. Take the following additional food supplements:
   - Wheat germ oil – 2 to 3 teaspoons a day.
   - Vitamin E – 300 to 600 I.U. a day (before meal). Note: in case of high blood pressure, consult your doctor for proper dosage of vitamin E.
   - Vitamin C (from a rose hips or other natural sources)– up to 1000 mg. a day.
   - Vitamin B-complex, high potency – one tablet a day.

- Cod liver oil, unfortified – 1 teaspoon a day.
- Vitamin A, natural – 25,000 USP units a day.
- Kelp – 10 tablets a day.
- Bone meal tablets, for minerals – 5 to 10 tablets a day.
- Cold–pressed vegetable oil, for vitamin F – 1 to 2 tablespoons a day. May be used on salads, cereals, etc. Olive oil, sunflower oil, soy oil, corn oil – all these oils are good for this purpose.

Where not suggested otherwise, food supplements should be taken with meals.

4. Do not overeat! Hardening of the arteries, which often accompanies obesity, may be a contributing cause of impaired blood circulation and diminished blood supply to your scalp.

5. Avoid alcohol, tobacco and salt. Avoid white sugar and white flour, and all products made with them.

6. Avoid excessive shampooing of your hair, unless your hair is excessively oily. The normal discharge of sebum, the oil from the sebaceous glands, is beneficial for your hair.

7. Vigorous brushing and finger or vibrator massage are extremely important for the healthy state of your hair and the prevention of baldness. Use a slant board or practice headstand regularly on a specially constructed stool (available at better health food stores) – both very effective in bringing more blood to blood-starving scalp.*

---

*See my booklet, STOP HAIR LOSS, for complete story of Dr. Engstrand's discovery as well as for the total program of nutritional and other means to improve hair growth and prevent baldness.

Chapter 14

Biological Medicine - The Healing Science of Tomorrow

The lay public tends to regard medical science and the current medical procedures and philosophies as something unimpeachable and indisputable. But just because a certain medical procedure or thinking is currently popular and is generally accepted in medical practice – or, in other words, is "orthodox" – does not mean that it will always be regarded as such. In medicine, ideas theories, methods and therapies come and go. Nor does the mere fact that a certain therapy is commonly accepted by orthodoxy, or is a part of traditional practice, guarantee that it is correct or even effective one. Tomorrow it may very well be regarded as a part of the ignorant or superstitious past. On the other hand, certain remedies and therapies which were scoffed at and regarded as quackery yesterday are viewed today with scientific respect and are incorporated into the arsenal of useful and accepted practice.

Throughout medical history, philosophies of the causes of disease and approved methods of healing have been changing almost with every generation. In just the last generation we have been witnessing numerous changes in medical thinking. For example:

- Hypnosis, regarded a generation ago as quackery, is now an accepted, respectable science.

- A generation ago, tonsils were routinely removed from babies as considered being unnecessary – now doctors realize that these organs have vital functions to perform.
- Prolonged bedrest after heart attacks or surgery or in general convalescence is now replaced with early ambulation.
- Vitamin E, which was regarded by F. D. A. just a decade ago as unnecessary in human nutrition, now is looked upon as a new wonder drug with near miraculous healing properties.

The rapid development of the chemical and physical sciences in the twentieth century has had a negative influence upon medical thinking and slowed the progress of medical science. Doctors have come to regard man as a chemo-physical conglomeration of separate parts. This thinking characterizes our era of specialization, where one doctor treats feet, another – skin, the third – eyes, the fourth – heart, and so on. These specialists are able neither to view disease as a disturbance of the entire organism, nor to treat it as such.

The fallacy of Pasteurian philosophy of disease

The twentieth century medical therapeutic methods are based on the Pasteurian assumption that diseases are caused by bacteria. Pasteur observed bacteria in disease and came to the conclusion that the bacteria were the *cause* of disease. Upon this fallacious conclusion western medical science has been based for the last 100 years. The medical science of twentieth century is aimed at protecting man from bacterial attack by pharmaceutical and surgical means.

In the last decade profound changes have been taking place in medical thinking. A growing number of progressive medical scientists, particularly in Europe, are moving from the Pasteurian concept of disease and symptomatic drug-therapy approach towards a new biological concept of medicine. Perhaps we should not speak of a *new* concept of thinking since truly there is "nothing new under the sun". Biological medicine is based on the teachings of the great Hippocrates, the "Father of Medicine", who two thousand years ago expounded that most, if not all, diseases are of man's own making and are the end result of a long-time abuse in the form of poor living habits, faulty nutrition and other health-destroying environmental factors. New medical thinking is directed toward a concept of a man as a whole entity with his physical and emotional aspects inseparably unified in one living soul. It sees man as an organic part of the biological and cosmic universe and subject to all the unchangeable and irrevocable laws of nature. Man's disregard of these laws in respect to his environment, nutrition and physical and emotional needs, leads to disharmony with the live-giving biological and spiritual universe. *Disease is a consequent result of this disharmony.*

Biological medicine is not a new philosophy or a passing fad. It is a true medical science based on the principle of intelligent support of the natural healing powers inherent in the living organism. Drugs never cure disease – at best they only suppress or alleviate the symptoms. Lasting results can be attained only when a wise doctor assists and supports the body's own healing forces, which institute the health-restoring processes and accomplish the actual cure. *Biological therapies are directed at correcting the underlying causes of disease, strengthening the patient's resistance and creating the most favorable conditions for the body's own healing processes to take place.*

Man's body is endowed with an enormous capacity to adapt itself to abnormal, adverse conditions. But this capacity is limited. When health-destroying conditions continue unchecked for prolonged periods of time, various disturbances in the functions of the organs and glands begin to manifest themselves. These may be in the form of fever, repeated colds and infections, tonsilitis, enlarged liver, increased blood pressure, skin eruptions, etc. In most instances these are protective and defensive measures initiated by the organism in its effort to protect itself against the existing abnormal conditions. Ignored or suppressed by drugs, such symptoms may get progressively worse or change their nature and ultimately result in chronic pathological and degenerative changes.

It is becoming increasingly evident that the present-day conventional drug-approach, which treats isolated symptoms, is unable to solve the problem of the catastrophic increase of the degenerative diseases, such as cancer, cardio-vascular disorders, arthritis, diabetes, etc. The conventional approach of treating specific symptoms with specific drugs or remedies, without taking into consideration the patient's total condition of health and correcting the underlying causes of his ill health, is as unscientific as it is ineffective. A more fundamental approach, which takes man's environmental factors, nutritional patterns and emotional attitudes into consideration, is long overdue. Biological medicine presents such an approach. Instead of the conventional masking of symptoms, biological treatments are directed toward the elimination of the basic causes of disease, helping the body's own healing activity and restoring the equilibrium and harmony in the functions of all its vital organs.

Dangers of conventional therapies

The conventional drug and surgery approach is associated with great risks and dangers. The alarming increase in iatrogenic (or doctor-induced) diseases, due to toxic drugs and needless or incompetently performed surgery, proves this. A recent six-year study conducted under direction of Dr. L. E. Cluff, professor of medicine at the University of Florida, reported to the U. S. Senate investigators that "adverse effects of non-prescription drugs as well as prescription drugs, are responsible for the hospitalization and death of a significant number of patients." It is estimated that at least ten per cent of all patients suffer from doctor caused diseases.

There is no such thing as a safe, harmless drug. All drugs, including common aspirin, are potentially dangerous. A study showed that some patients get 10 to 12 different drugs, some as many as 42 at the same time. No wonder that drug illnesses involving medical service is the *seventh most common cause of hospitalization in the United States.*

The list of new drugs available to the present-day physician is growing faster than the average doctor has time to learn about their properties or potential dangers. He has to depend on the subjective and often exaggerated claims of drug manufacturers, which usually overestimate the benefits and underestimate the dangers of their drugs. Seventy per cent of all prescriptions filled in 1963 were for drugs introduced since 1950. This shows that thousands of drugs used prior to 1950, including many of the "wonder" and "miracle" drugs, have been discontinued as either ineffective or too dangerous to use. Many wonder drugs in current use may be potential killers, as all too frequently is discovered – unfortunately, only after many patients have paid with their lives for their doctor's experiments. Just recently, a medical investigation accused the Food and Drug Administration of licensing a drug, *indomethacin,* labeled as a "wonder drug" for the treatment of rheumatoid arthritis, and permitting its use for several years. The drug had caused severe reactions in patients and many deaths. The manufacturers claimed it was relatively nontoxic, but the drug caused peptic ulcers, lesions in small bowels, severe headaches to the point that some patients became psychotic, and some deaths.

Another "wonder" drug, *chloromycetin,* a potent antibiotic, the use of which is supposed to be restricted to only a few serious diseases, such as typhoid fever, but in fact has been even prescribed for colds and minor infections, was found to be lethally dangerous. Several "horrid" deaths, due to aplastic anemia which the drug causes, have been reported. "It is hardly conceivable that this has been going on for 18 years", said Dr. Franklin Farman of Lakewood, California, to the U.S. Senate Small Business Monopoly Subcommittee.

Even such a simple drug as *aspirin,* believed by most people to be completely harmless, and used massively by Americans, adults and children alike – at the rate of 49 tons a day! – is potentially a very dangerous drug, implicated in an increasing number of ill effects, such as severe asthma, kidney disease, pathological changes in the liver, gastric hemorrhage, cell-shedding and consequent erosion of the lining of the stomach, blood disorders, cardiac weakness, albuminuria, inflammation of nasal passages, and nasal polyps. Aspirin is also known as a vitamin antagonist. It is especially devastating to vitamin C and destroys hughe quantities of it in the body. And, very recently, medical researchers, Dr. N. Neal Pinckard, et al., have found that aspirin "profoundly changes the structure of the blood plasma" and may effect a "wide variety of physiological and pathological changes". In view of aspirin's "widespread and indiscriminate" use they asked for serious investigation of its potential dangers.

X-rays are used indiscriminately on a wide scale, especially by dentists. American dentists now refuse to extract a tooth or fix a cavity without an X-ray. And they insist that their regular patients take routine X-rays *twice a year* from every angle, just to see if any new cavities are developing. This is in spite of the well-known fact that the harmful effects of X-rays are cumulative and that more and more evidence is turning up which puts irradiation by X-rays as a suspect in many diseases, including cancer and leukemia. Recent studies made under a Public Health Service grant show that irradiation of the mother before conception and irradiation of the mother during pregnancy are associated with the later development of leukemia in the child.

Biological therapies 100% safe

Biological treatments, on the other hand, are completely safe and harmless. The arsenal of biological therapies includes dietetic restriction, controlled fasting, juice therapies, hydrotherapies, heat therapies, special exercises, massage and physiotherapy, herb preparations, vitamin-mineral-trace-element supplementation, and special biological medicines made from organic and inorganic substances found in nature and prepared in accordance with biological principles. These medicines are never synthetic and are completely non-toxic. Several drug companies in Europe specialize in production of such preparations, notably WELEDA and WALA in Switzerland. These preparations are administered both orally and as subcutaneous injections. All the biological therapies, including biological medication, are free from undesired side-effects and they do not alter nor interfere with normal functions of the organs or in the metabolic processes – only support and activate them. They stimulate the glands and other vital organs of the body and accelerate the healing processes.

What is biological medicine?

I presented this question to Dr. Lars-Erik Essén, M. D., the foremost representative of biological medicine in Sweden and the leading spirit behind the new and growing movement of progressive doctors who follow the principles of biological medicine in their practice.

"May I, instead of using dry, scientific definitions, illuminate this with a concrete example?" said Dr. Essén. "A doctor is treating a case of infectious disease by the conventional methods. The determining factor for a successful result of this kind of treatment is to identify the kind of bacteria considered responsible for the infection in question. When the intruder is identified, the patient is given a specific chemical or antibiotic drug, which, as a rule, accomplishes the immediate results: the bacteria are destroyed and the patient is free from symptoms.

"After a while, it may happen that the same patient will turn up with a new infection. The diagnosis shows that either it is a question of the same kind of bacteria, which this time, however, is already immune to the specific drug, or that there are new bacteria involved. Accordingly, new and more potent drugs are prescribed, which bring about immediate results, as far as fighting the bacteria is concerned. But in spite of the 'success' of the treatment, the patient's resistance to infection seems to weaken progressively and various complications set in. Now, perhaps, such potent drugs as cortisone – pain-killer and symptom-reliever – and other highly toxic synthetic drugs enter the picture. The body, already weakened by the disease, must now, in addition, cope with the toxic and damaging side effects of the poisonous drugs.

"Then, one day, we stand by the deathbed surprised and shocked. The patient had received all the correct treatments in accordance with medical science's conventional practices and regulations. The laboratory tests proved that we made no errors! Bacteria samples showed that the bacteria, which our treatment was aimed at, were "successfully" eradicated. As far as the direct cause of the symptoms was concerned (the bacteria) our treatment was a complete success. The only problem was that the patient died! We succeeded in killing the bacteria, but we failed to save the host organism, where our war on bacteria was so successful. It also could be said that 'The operation was successful, but the patient didn't survive.'

"Now, actually, this kind of a result is not so surprising, is it?" continued Dr. Essén. "After all, what did we treat? Our treatment was directed at micro-organisms which we considered pathogenic or disease-causing. In the meantime, the biological environment for this micro-organism, the host organism, the living, delicate, sensitive, and easily-damaged human body, has actually been completely neglected. The man hardly comes into the picture at all. What we actually treat today are diseases, not the diseased people. The sick body, however, is subject to very different biological laws than those which could be applied in a primitive germ war with chemical and antibiotic germ-killers.

"A parallel to this can be seen in today's damage and destruction of life and natural environment as a result of man's indiscriminate use of insecticides and other poisonous chemicals. Is there any intelligent human being who is so naïve as to assume that these poisons will be less devastating to the human body, with its endlessly more intricate and delicate living mechanism? The biological laws of life are quite different from the laws which regulate chemical reactions observed in laboratory tubes. When we fail to see the differences between the two, catastrophic conditions will be the result, and we have to accept the consequences of our unwise actions."

Philosophy of Biological Medicine

"When the biologically oriented physician is confronted with a case of infectious disease his approach and his actions are entirely different. For him, bacteria and viruses which are present in certain infections, are phenomena of secondary interest. He considers them only as symptomatic factors in relation to the host organism (the patient) and his body as a biological environment. All his attention is directed towards the patient. His primary aim is to employ every measure available to increase the power of resistance within the host organism and avoid causing it any damage. The first principle of the art of healing, 'Primum est nil nocere' – the most important thing of all is that the treatment must do no harm – is violated in present-day medical practice more than in any other period or medical history.

"The biologically oriented doctor is aware that with chemical and antibiotic drugs he will always cause damage to the host organism's biological milieu, even though with such treatments he can achieve a temporary effect. Therefore, he avoids to the utmost the use of such drugs in the management of simple and harmless infections. To treat a common cold or a sore throat with, for example, penicillin, for him is a crime against the fundamental rules of health. Instead, his attention is directed to increasing the body's own resistance with all the natural, harmless, biological methods of treatment which are now available."

The point of no return

"The catastrophic point of no return to which chemically and technologically oriented medicine has evolved, has given basis for new medical thinking: biological medicine. Its assertion is that the physical-chemical laws can not be indiscriminately applied on the biological reality, with its multiplicity of distinctive and unique characteristics, without assaulting the objective criteria of the reality one is trying to serve. The biological phenomena are not subordinated to the physical-chemical laws – they are, on the contrary, superior to them. While conventional, orthodox medicine considers that chemical substances can substitute for the biological processes, biological medicine rejects such thinking as a form of modern superstition. The biological processes can only be understood in their unique peculiarity. The pathological abnormalities in the biological processes can only be corrected by changes in the biological environment. Bacteria or virus are not primary causes of disease; they are only symptomatic factors of the biological milieu. To correct this milieu is of the utmost importance for the successful management of disease. Chemical drugs can, at their best, serve only for the temporary relief of symptoms. Prolonged use of drugs will always damage the biological milieu. The normalizing of this milieu, or creating of the biological environment most conducive for the healing processes, is the prime goal of the biologically oriented physician.

"Many patients have been restored to health through the practiced application of biological medicine after all the conventional treatments have failed. Biological medicine and naturopathic methods of treatment will come to the fore more and more as the successful alternative to conventional therapy; and for the afflicted, who tried in vain conventional therapy, they present the only choice. The philosophy of biological medicine is not in opposition to conventional medicine; it rather widens, deepens and complements it."*

Biological medicine is based on the following basic premises:

1. Most chronic, degenerative diseases, as well as the most infectious and inflammatory conditions are caused by metabolic disorders and systemic disturbances which are in turn brought about by the pathological biochemical changes in the tissues and organs of the body.

2. The underlying causes for these systemic disturbances and pathological changes are to be sought in the prolonged abuses to which the body has been subjected, such as faulty nutritional patterns, overeating, nutritional deficiencies, chronic poisoning by the chemical additives and residues in food, air and water,

---

*The quote taken from the Foreword of my book, THERE IS A CURE FOR ARTHRITIS, written by Dr. Lars-Erik Essén, M.D.

drug poisoning, lack of sufficient rest and exercise, severe emotional and physical stresses, etc. These health-destroying environmental factors eventually result in diminished vitality and lowered resistance to disease, biochemical imbalance, disordered metabolism, impaired elimination and autointoxication.

3. Biological treatments are aimed, therefore, at the eradication and the correction of all the abnormal health-destroying conditions that have lead to the development of the disease. This usually begins with a total withdrawal of drugs; radical changes in eating habits with emphasis on fresh raw fruits and vegetables; exclusion of sugar, alcohol, coffee, tea, soda drinks, tobacco, salt, white flour and all the products made from it (cakes, pastries, refined cereals, etc.); controlled fasting and juice therapy; therapeutic baths and other hydrotherapy; etc.

4. Biological treatments are directed towards normalizing metabolic processes, establishing biochemical stability, strengthening the functions of vital organs, revitalizing glandular activity, re-establishing capillary integrity, and, in general, rebuilding and strengthening the general health of the patient.

5. The ultimate goal of biological treatments is to help the defensive and healing powers of the body in their constant effort to counteract health-destroying influences, correct existing disturbances, bring about necessary repair and effect the actual cure. *Thus, the cure is always accomplished by the body's own curative forces – biological therapies only eliminate the causative factors, strengthen the body and stimulate and assist its restorative and healing activity.*

Conventional versus biological medicine

From the above it can be easily seen why some modern doctors, who look upon their profession as a business, would not be very interested in biological medicine. It is a time-consuming and tedious job to try to discover the initial causative factors of the ill health of each patient, then convince and instruct him in necessary changes in his environment, diet, living habits, etc., and help to rebuild and strengthen his total health. It is much faster, just a matter of a few minutes, to write a prescription for a drug, which will temporarily suppress the unwanted symptoms and make the patient feel that he has really been helped.

There is, however, an important difference between these two diagnostic and therapeutic procedures, the conventional drug approach and the biological medical approach. While in the former case the patient will be back in a short while with some other or similar symptoms, in the latter case the treatment will bring the total and the lasting removal and correction of the existing diseased conditions.

Biological medicine – the healing science of tomorrow

The healing science of today is in a state of utter chaos. The orthodox, allopathic medicine, misdirected by the fallacious Pasteurian concept of disease and consequently relying on drugs and surgery in its effort to conquer illness, has entered a viscious cycle. The complete fiasco of today's medicine is evidenced by the fact that in spite of more doctors, more hospitals, and more money spent on health than at any time in man's history (more than 60 billion dollars a year!), we have more disease than ever before. And we are witnessing a catastrophic increase in all the chronic degenerative conditions including heart disease and cancer. Already *one half* of the American people are chronically ill. Our mortality rate is increasing – it is now about 50th among the world's nations. And our life expectancy is going down. We occupy 18th place for men and 11th place for women in life expectancy among industrialized nations.

Because of the medical doctors' inability to reverse the trend, people are losing their faith in them. So-called fringe medicines are blooming as never before. The sick people, not finding relief in drugs, are going to chiropractors, osteopaths, naturopaths, spiritual healers, physiotherapists, herbalists, nutritionists, drugless healers, Christian Scientists, etc. Or they take their health into their own hands and try to improve it with better nutrition, health foods, food supplements, vitamins, and exercise. Fearing the rapidly approaching end of its monopoly in the healing arts, the orthodoxy is fighting back fiercely trying to make fringe medicines unlawful and by enacting laws that would make selling health foods and vitamins illegal. Today's medical history is full of persistent intolerence on the part of orthodox practitioners, and of violent opposition to and persecution of unorthodox philosophies and unconventional healing methods. Many practitioners using unorthodox methods of healing have been thrown into jails, just like in the time of the dark ages.

The totalitarian and relentless methods with which orthodox medicine tries to save its crumbling empire can result only in the total loss of the people's confidence and respect and in the inevitable final crash. On the ruins of the crumbled orthodoxy, destroyed by conceit, intolerance and greed, a new kind of medicine will be born – biological medicine, the medical science of tomorrow.

Biological medicine is not opposed to *any* of the healing systems, including the medical. Its philosophy is based on the fundamental principle of intelligent cooperation with nature. It sees man as a part of nature, subject to its eternal laws. It is a modern science which incorporates all the harmless and effective therapies that can be applied in the correction of diseases and restoration of health.

Tomorrow's doctors of biological medicine will be trained in all the known arts of healing: allopathic, naturopathic, chiropractic, herbal, homeopathic, psychosomatic, spiritual, etc. The biological doctor will recognize that no doctor and no remedy can cure disease. Disease can be cured only by the body's own inherent healing power. Biological doctor will assist these healing forces and create the most favorable conditions for the healing processes to take place. All known supportive therapeutic methods will be available for his use. Where life can be saved with drugs, they will be employed. Where surgery is needed because of accidents of other causes, it will be used. Where there is damage or dislocation in the spine or the joints – then chiropractic treatments will be applied. Where the disease is caused by systemic disorders and biochemical imbalance due to faulty eating and living habits – the corrective nutrition and naturopathic healing methods will be used. Where the condition is caused by mental stress, or other psychic causes, spiritual healing, and psychological approaches can be used.

Tomorrow's doctor of biological medicine will be a true doctor – which means teacher. He will teach people the correct ways of eating and living so that they can avoid ever becoming sick. Biological medicine will stress the preventive approach to disease. "An ounce of prevention is worth a pound of cure" will become the norm, rather than an empty phrase.

Biological medicine is the perfect science of healing of which Hippocrates dreamed. When its precepts are accepted by all practitioners of the healing arts and applied in the management of man's ills, then, and only then, the diseased mankind will be freed from the dark inferno of modern pestilence and plague into which he has been thrust by the misdirected chemical, pharamacological and medical sciences.

A new era of glorious, buoyant health and a total freedom from disease will emerge. Man will live in peace and harmony with nature, with animals and, last but not least – with his neighbors. The healthy body and mind will constitute a worthy temple for the spirit to dwell in. Freed from disease and pain, man will be able to pursue his true purpose in life – the perfection of his human and divine characteristics and the refinement of his spirit.

Chapter 15

Questions and Answers

During the question and answer periods after my lectures I receive hundreds of questions from the audience. Some of these are of a personal nature, of course, but most are of a general character, the answers to which would interest most readers. It has been during these question and answer periods that I have become acutely aware of appalling confusion regarding the most elementary and basic issues of nutrition – even among those who had read, studied and applied nutrition for years. The most common questions concern protein needs, vitamin supplements, man's ideal diet, vegetarianism, fasting, bread, milk, and inorganic minerals. These questions are answered in detail in the respective chapters of this book. Here are a few other frequently asked questions and answers:

VITAMINS

Q. *Can vitamins in large doses be harmful?*

A. As a rule, vitamins, even in very large doses, are completely harmless. There is a notable exception, however: large doses of some isolated synthetic vitamins, particularly isolated vitamins of the B-complex, and vitamins A and D. These vitamins should not be taken in synthetic form in large doses without expert professional advice. Of course, there is no risk involved even with these vitamins if they are taken in the form of brewer's yeast (for B-vitamins) and unfortified fish liver oils (for A and D).

It is wisest and safest to take vitamins and minerals in the form of food supplements, where they occur in their natural form and strength, and in combination with all the other nutritive factors such as enzymes and trace elements, for optimum assimilation and biological activity. Vitamins in food supplements are perfectly harmless.

VITAMIN B_{15}

Q. *We hear so much about vitamin B_{15} lately, about its remarkable benefits. Why is it beneficial, and if it is as beneficial as it is claimed to be, why then FDA has banned its sale in the United States?*

A. The latter part of your question must be answered by the FDA. They have banned, or were trying to ban, many other beneficial vitamins and nutritive substances, such as Bioflavonoids, or vitamin P, for instance.

Vitamin B_{15}, or pangamic acid, is one of the B-complex vitamins. Most of research on vitamin B_{15} comes from Russia, although it was discovered in the United States by Dr. E. T. Krebs and his associates. A team of Russian researchers have discovered that "vitamin B_{15} increases general and myocardial resistance to hypoxia". Hypoxia means an insufficient supply of oxygen to the living tissues.

The discovery has great importance and wide application in medicine. An insufficient supply of oxygen to the tissues is linked with such serious conditions as heart disease, anemia, acute poisonings, etc. Many scientists (Warburg, Goldblatt, et al.) believe that a periodic lack of oxygen must be held responsible for the formation of cancer cells, thus being one of the causes of cancer.

One of our gravest health problems today is a chronic poisoning by carbon monoxide from the polluted air which covers most of our larger cities. Carbon monoxide induces hypoxia by preventing oxygen from being absorbed by the lungs. If vitamin B_{15} can increase the body's resistance to hypoxia, or lack of oxygen, then it can help us to protect ourselves against slow poisoning by carbon monoxide, to which we are all subjected.

It is believed that the American diet is generally deficient in vitamin B_{15}. It occurs naturally in whole grains and seeds, brewer's yeast, brown rice and rice polishings. Sunflower, pumpkin and sesame seeds are good sources of this vitamin.

SALT

Q. *There is so much controversy on the salt question. Is salt a poison as some authorities suggest, or is it a necessary substance in good nutrition?*

A. To say that salt is poison is to tell only a half-truth. Your body needs salt, or sodium chloride, for its many important metabolic functions – among other things, for the hydrochloric acid production in the stomach. Reliable studies show that your daily need of salt is between 0.2 and 0.6 grams a day. This amount of salt can be easily obtained from the foods you eat, provided you eat predominantly raw natural foods. Cooking in water removes salt and other minerals from the foods.

Civilized man takes far too much table salt with his food. The animal protein foods and other overcooked foods he eats are not palatable without large amounts of salt. Many people eat as much as 10 to 15 grams of salt every day. In such amounts salt definitely is a poison within the body. Too much salt may cause such disorders as kidney problems, heart and blood vessel conditions, high blood pressure, rheumatic diseases, hair loss, and skin disorders. Research has revealed that your kidneys are capable of eliminating up to five grams of salt per day. Salt consumed above this amount will have to remain in the body. But in its concentrated form it can cause damage; so your body has to store it in its various organs and tissues in solution of 1 part of salt to 20 parts of water. Edema is usually nothing but stored salt water that overworked kidneys or skin are not able to excrete.

Salt metabolism is one of the most misunderstood body processes – by the layman as well as by the learned. You have been told that when you sweat a lot from physical exertion or high temperature, you *lose* lots of salt through the perspiration. And you have also been told that this lost salt *must be replaced,* or you will have a salt deficiency. This is the most nonsensical theory on a body function I have ever heard – and I have heard quite a few nonsensical theories. To say that your body loses salt, *which it needs,* with sweat, is to display total ignorance of the body's inherent wisdom. The truth is, in fact, exactly the opposite: *your body uses perspiration as a welcomed opportunity to get rid of the undesirable, toxic salt from its tissues.* To replace this salt, after your body has succeeded in excreting it with perspiration, is to do your body a great disservice.

Do not forget that your skin is your biggest eliminative organ, "the third kidney". When your kidneys are overloaded and can not successfully detoxify your blood from all the present toxins, the skin takes over and helps the kidneys to eliminate the undesirable substances. Thus, salt, uric acid, purines and other toxins are thrown out with the sweat.

To suggest that you have to eat more salt when you "lose" it in perspiration is not a more logical deduction than to suggest that you have to eat more sugar when your body is "losing" it through the urine, as in the case of diabetes.

Your body does not need salt to perspire; it can perspire without it. I haven't used any salt to speak of for twenty-five years. I exercise and work very hard, run several miles each day, use a sauna once or twice a week – and sweat profusely. Often I spend several months in tropical heat and perspire gallons of water each day. My perspiration has no salty taste, and I have never experienced symptoms of salt deficiency. On occasions when I consumed salt unknowingly, however, I could taste it the next day in my perspiration.

In an optimum diet for optimum health salt should be kept to a minimum. If some addition of salt is desired, small amounts of sea salt could be used. Kelp is also an excellent substitute for salt. Kelp granules or powder can be used as a flavoring in cooking, sprinkled over salads, etc.

FERMENTED FOODS

Q. *Europeans eat lots of fermented foods, such as sauerkraut, sour pickles, sour bread, sour milk, etc. What nutritional advantage does sour foods have, if any?*

A. All peoples known for their exceptionally good health and long life use lots of fermented foods in their diet – Hunzas, Bulgarians, Germans, Russians. Bulgarians eat sour milk, sour vegetables and sour bread. Sauerkraut is an important part of the German diet. Black sour bread is Russia's staple; the average Russian eats 2 pounds of it a day.

Fermented foods have been used not only as a food, but also as a medicine. Miraculous cures from arthritis, scurvy, ulcers, colds, digestive disorders, even cancer, have been attributed to the regular use of fermented foods. People have eaten these foods for centuries without knowing why they had such a curative effect. Now, German cancer researcher, Dr. Johannes Kuhl, shed some light on this question. He explains the healing property of fermented foods thus:

"Natural lactic acid and fermentive enzymes, which are produced during the fermentation process, have a beneficial effect on metabolism and a curative effect on disease."

Lactic acid destroys harmful intestinal bacteria and contributes to the better digestion and assimilation of nutrients. Fermented foods can be considered pre-digested foods, very easily digested and assimilated, even by persons with weak digestive organs. Fermented foods improve intestinal hygiene and provide a proper environment for the body's own vitamin production within the intestines. They are excellent preventive foods against constipation.

Warning: do not use commercial sauerkraut or sour pickles

from your supermarket. They are prepared with vinegars and can not be considered natural lactic acid foods. Make your own fermented foods (see recipes for sour bread, sour milk, sauerkraut, and sour pickles in Chapter 16 of this book) or buy natural lactic acid foods at your health food store.

YOGURT

Q. *What about yogurt-cataract scare?*

A. Some anti-yogurt (read: anti-health) forces created a worldwide scare in August 1970 by reporting that feeding yogurt to rats resulted in cataracts in a large percentage of the rats. A milk sugar substance, *galactose,* found in yogurt, was blamed for the cataracts in rats. Many regular users of yogurt stopped eating this wonder food, since the news was widely publicised in all news media, and it was implied that yogurt may also produce cataracts on humans.

There is no scientific basis for such an assumption, however. Here are a few facts to consider:

1. Rats in reported cases were fed yogurt *exclusively* for most of their lives. No human being ever subsisted on yogurt alone. Dr. Frank W. Newell, head of Ophthalmology Department of Chicago University, said: "No human being could possibly consume enough galactose in a lifetime to produce cataracts."

2. Dr. Ed Cotlier, Assistant Professor of Ophthalmology at the University of Illinois, states: "The metabolic system of the rat is different from man's. Rats are deficient in an enzyme that brakes down galactose into nutrients. Man has this enzyme in the liver."

3. There is not a single case known where cataracts were caused in humans by eating yogurt.

In view of the above facts and the authoritive statements by eminent scientists, it would be foolsih to curtail in the slightest, the consumption of yogurt – one of our real wonder foods. The whole cataract-scare incident could be summed with the words of Stephen Gaymont, President of Gaymont Laboratories in Chicago, who called the theory "an idiotic claim with no foundation."

CELL SALTS

Q. *What is the value of cell salts?*

A. Cell salts is a new fad. But there is nothing new about cell salts. They are good old homeopathic pills, known and used for a century, but resurrected from the dusty homeopathic pharmacy shelves. They contain all the basic minerals from which our body is built. Like all homeopathic drugs, cell salts are reduced to extremely low potencies by the process called trituration.

The amount of minerals received by taking homeopathic remedies is so small that they can not be considered as food supplements or nutrients. The therapeutic effect of homeopathic remedies is based on the totally different principle: they act as stimulants which increase the body's ability to assimilate nutrients from foods.

As with all medication, cell salts should be used according to the advice of homeopathic physicians who can diagnose the condition and prescribe the proper remedies. You will find the names of homeopathic doctors and pharmacies in the Yellow Pages of your telephone book.

NUTRITION AND SEX

Q. *What is the truth about nutritional aphrodisiacs? Is it true that some foods can increase virility and sexual power?*

A. There is a growing conviction among clinical nutritionists and doctors that many sexual inadequacies and disorders, such as male impotency, female frigidity, male and female sterility, premature abortions, menstrual pains and menopausal distress, have nutritional origins. Throughout the history of mankind there has existed a widespread and persistent conviction that there is an unmistakable relationship between man's nutrition and his physical capacity for love, as evidenced by countless ancient medical records, scriptures, folklore and tradition. Modern medical science has always derided this idea as sheer nonsense and superstition.

In the last few decades we have been experiencing a sexual revolution. The chains of taboos and inhibitions are being broken. Sex has become a legitimate subject for scientific inquiry. Although most of the scientific studies so far approach the subject from the psychological and sociological viewpoint, there is a steadily growing number of researchers who are delving into the physiological and the biological aspects of sex. Nutrition is coming into the limelight as a vitally important factor affecting man's sexual life.

The scientific studies of nutrition as related to man's sexual life and his virility demonstrate that there is a *definite relationship* between man's sexual health and vigor and the food he eats.

In addition to the fact that good nutrition in general is essential for man's health and for the healthy function of the reproductive organs, there are certain particular foods and food substances which have a direct beneficial effect on the sex glands. Sex glands need specific nutrients, minerals, vitamins and natural chemicals, in order to function properly. For example, the mineral zinc has been found to be absolutely essential for the health of the prostate gland. Vitamin B_1, vitamins A and E, and lecithin are involved directly and indirectly in stimulating and enhancing the proper function of the sexual glands and increasing the sex hormone production. Vitamin E particularly is of paramount importance for sexual health. Foods that contain these special nutrients can be called nutritional aphrodisiacs.

In my book, SEX AND NUTRITION, which is a modern scientific study on nutritional aspects of sexuality, both male and female, I list 10 special foods and food substances that have a particularly beneficial effect in maintaining and enhancing sexual vigor. These foods are excellent sources of nutrition needed for the healthy functioning of the endocrine and sex glands. They are completely natural and harmless. They are not artificial stimulants that overstimulate the sexual glands into unnatural activity or endanger health, but are foods that will help the glands to reach the peak of healthy activity. The ten special foods are: *wheat germ, wheat germ oil, lecithin, milk, honey, eggs, sesame seeds, kelp, fish liver oil and raw nuts and seeds.* The first three are relatively new foods, but the others are foods that have been used by men and women for thousands of years for the purpose of enhancing their amatory prowess. They are named and recommended in many ancient writings and their reputations are time-tested.

These ten special foods have been proven by the modern science of nutrition and/or by extended empirical evidence to have a beneficial stimulating effect on the healthy activity of the endocrine and sex glands and, thus, they hold a recognized potential for improved sexual vigor and health.

For detailed instructions on how to use these foods, a complete description of their nutritive values, and the scientific justification for their use as nutritional aphrodisiacs, see my book, *SEX AND NUTRITION.* *

JOGGING

Q. *There has been a great deal of controversy recently in regard to jogging; What is your opinion?*

A. Today's soft, sedentary living is one of the main causes of our physical deterioration. There is ample medical evidence that lots of physical exercise is imperative for optimum health. Walking, with intermittent slow jogging, outdoors in fresh air, is the best form of exercise for any age.

Jogging, a recent import from Australia, has swept the nation in just a couple of years. Only a few years ago, however, it was such an unusual activity that every time I jogged in the streets in the United States, a police patrolman or regular driver would stop to give me a ride, thinking that the poor man was in a hurry to get somewhere. But now, a man jogging along the streets is an integral part of American life.

But, another integral part of American life is the *contradictory information,* so even this issue is confused. I have spoken in favor of jogging, but there are opinions against it as well. Some doctors

---

*Paavo O. Airola, SEX AND NUTRITION, Information Incorporated, New York, 1970.

have expressed warnings that jogging is a dangerous fad, that it can cripple and even kill.

First, do not confuse *jogging* with *running.* The correct way to jog is to make almost-on-the-spot running, moving forward very slowly, not faster than ordinary walking. Two people jogging side by side should be able to have a relaxed conversation without experiencing shortness of breath. Such jogging is hardly more tiring than regular walking. But it is far more beneficial, because it sets in motion virtually all the muscles of the body and stimulates all the organs and glands. It also produces greater tissue oxygenation.

Jogging should be introduced gradually. Start with short periods of jogging during your regular walking; one-half to one minute periods are sufficient. Increase the time gradually. As soon as you feel tired or short of breath, stop jogging and walk slowly. *Note:* never jog – or walk – on busily trafficked streets, if you don't want to be fumigated to death. If you live in the city, drive out to the countryside where there is fresh, clean air, and jog there.

Jogging is a perfectly safe form of exercise, if done properly. Even old people, including so-called heart cases, can jog slowly and for short periods. The key word is *moderation;* do not overdo. Never jog when tired, on smoggy city streets or right after a meal.

GARLIC AND ONIONS

Q. *Are garlic and onions health foods, or are they harmful, as some health writers suggest?*

A. Garlic and onions are among the most important "wonder" health foods. Garlic is "king" and onion is "queen" of the vegetable kingdom. Both have been used for thousands of years as food and as medicine. Miraculous healing powers seem to exist in both. Babylonians used garlic to cure many diseases as early as 3,000 B.C. Chinese, Greeks, Romans, Egyptians, Hindus, Vikings – all have used garlic to cure everything from intestinal disorders to the symptoms of premature aging. The great ancient physicians – Aristophanes, Pliny, Dioscorides, Hippocrates, Galen, Paracelsus – prescribed garlic for a variety of disorders.

Modern research has confirmed that garlic and onions do indeed possess miracle healing powers. Russian electrobiologist, Professor Gurwitch, discovered that garlic and onions emit a peculiar type of ultra-violet radiation called mitogenetic radiations. These radiations – the Gurwitch rays – have the property of stimulating cell growth and activity, and have a rejuvenating effect on all body functions. A great amount of scientific research has been done in various countries on the therapeutic properties of garlic and onions. Dr. A. I. Virtanen, Finnish Nobel Prize Winner, discovered 14 new beneficial substances in onions. German, French, English, American and Russian researchers have used garlic on thousands of patients and concluded that it is indeed a miracle medicinal food. It has been successfully used to treat the following conditions: high or low blood pressure, common colds, intestinal worms, coughs, asthma, whooping cough, intestinal putrefaction, dysentery, gastrointestinal disorders, gas, tuberculosis, and diabetes. American research has shown that garlic is a powerful agent against tumor formation in cancer. It also has been found to be an effective agent in preventing diphtheria, typhus, and pneumonia. Russians discovered that garlic has antibiotic properties; they even refer to garlic as *Russian penicillin.* Russian medical clinics and hospitals use garlic extensively, mostly in the form of volatile extracts that are vaporized and inhaled.

I have used garlic very successfully to treat patients with diarrhea, intestinal putrefaction, gas, asthma and high blood pressure. In some cases, the blood pressure was reduced 20 to 30 mm. in one week by taking large amounts of garlic.

In addition to having such miraculous healing qualities, garlic and onions are most delicious foods. Used wisely, they can improve the taste of many dishes and salads.

I only wish someone would discover an effective garlic-breath and onion-breath remover, so that we all could enjoy these miracle healing plants without social limitations! Odorless garlic pills?

I have tried many brands but haven't found one yet that does what it promises. Eating parsley and other chlorophyll-rich vegetables helps, but it does not remove the odor completely. So the only solution seems to be that either we all eat garlic, or those of us who do eat it move to Italy where everyone eats it all the time!

SUN BATHING

Q. *I'd love to get a good tan, but hate to get skin cancer. What should I do?*

A. The public has been made to believe that sun bathing is a very dangerous fad which can result in serious conditions, including sunstroke and skin cancer. Actually, the dangers of sun bathing are overemphasized. Naturally, sun bathing – as well as anything else – should be done in moderation. The skin has to be conditioned to sunshine. The tan that protects the body from overexposure must be built gradually. The best time to take a sun bath is before 11 AM or after 3 PM, when the rays are less harsh. Bathe only 15 minutes the first day, and add 15 more minutes a day until a good tan is produced.

In addition to giving a beautiful tan, sun bathing, or heliotherapy, is extremely beneficial therapeutic agent. Many serious diseases have been treated successfully by sunlight – tuberculosis, rickets, anemia, nervous disorders, respiratory disorders, rheumatic and arthritic conditions, psoriasis, obesity, circulatory disorders, glandular inactivity, etc. Sun is a tonic and stimulant, an invigorator and rejuvenator. It revitalizes the functioning of every gland in your body.

Vitamin D is produced on your skin by the effect of sun rays, then absorbed into your body. Vitamin D is particularly needed for the proper assimilation of minerals.

Used properly and in moderation – but year around – sun bathing is perfectly safe. Constant exposure to the powerful solar energy is an absolute necessity for vibrant health – indeed, for life itself. Plants, animals or man can not live long if totally deprived of the life-giving and healing rays of the sun.

Always remember, however, that the sun should be treated with respect. It is always wise to protect your head from its burning rays, and not to sun bathe during the middle of the day. Any signs of peeling or blisters indicate that you over-exposed yourself. Again, the sun, like any other good thing, should be used with moderation.

APPLE CIDER VINEGAR

Q. *Is apple cider vinegar a cure-all, or is its value overestimated?*

A. Dr. D. C. Jarvis, M. D., has made apple cider vinegar and honey popular in this country. A simple drink of two teaspoonfuls of apple cider vinegar and two teaspoonfuls of honey in a glass of water taken at each meal is supposed to cure practically every ill of mankind.

Honey is, of course, a real miracle food as well as one of man's oldest medicines. Both nutritional and therapeutic values of honey are so great that it is universally accepted as a must in any nutritional plan for optimum health, long life and prevention of disease.

Most people of middle age and over usually experience diminished secretion of hydrochloric acid in their stomach. Hydrochloric acid is needed for the digestion of protein-rich foods, and for the proper absorption of minerals and water-soluble vitamins B and C. In addition, hydrochloric acid acts as a natural disinfectant; it kills all pathogenic bacteria which enter the stomach via foods and drinks. The scientific motivation, therefore, for taking apple cider vinegar is based on the assumption that it helps to compensate for insufficient secretion of hydrochloric acid and, thus, improves the digestion and assimilation of foods.

Whether or not apple cider vinegar can actually substitute for hydrochloric acid in the stomach and perform the same functions, is not known. But it does create an acid condition in the stomach and digestive tract, which is important for good digestion and assimilation of foods. Of course, other fruit acids, such as lemon or lime juice and pineapple juice, taken with meals, will have about the same effect. The Mexican custom of spicing virtually all foods with lime juice is the Southern equivalent to Vermont's apple cider vinegar custom.

Warning: ordinary white vinegar is not suitable for these purposes and should never be used. Natural apple cider vinegar is sold in health food stores.

HYDROCHLORIC ACID

Q. *Is it advisable to take hydrochloric acid tablets as a digestive aid?*

A. I have seen quite dramatic improvements in some older people when they begin to take hydrochloric acid tablets after each meal. But your doctor should determine whether or not your hydrochloric acid secretion is sufficient.

Hydrochloric acid tablets are good preventive – and cure – for common dysentery, or what is called in Mexico *"turista"*. I have seen many cases of "turista" clear up in just a few days when the patient was permitted only cooked foods, mostly rice and applesauce, and given 1 hydrochloric acid tablet with each meal. Those American tourists who take hydrochloric acid tablets each day merely as a precautionary measure usually escape "turista" completely.

Hydrochloric acid in 3% solution can also be used for washing vegetables and fruits. It destroys pathogenic bacteria and removes pesticide residues. Produce should be left in the solution for 5 minutes, then rinsed in pure water.

REJUVENATING HERBS

Q. *What is all this excitement about the rejuvenating properties of Ginseng, Fo-ti-Tieng, Gotu-Kola, Damiana, etc? Do they really work?*

A. Throughout the ages man has used his inventive faculty to find ways of prolonging life, and particularly of rejuvenating his aging body and mind. Herbs have been used in every land and by every race as healing and rejuvenating agents since the very beginning of man's existence. The earliest medical writings, dating as far back as 5000 years, recommended thousands of herbs for medicinal use.

Twentieth century medicine, bumptiously blinded by the rapid advance of chemical science, has branded herbal medicines and rejuvenators remnants of an ignorant, superstitious past. "Nature" and "herbs" have become dirty words in modern medical vocabulary. Natural medicines have been replaced by the coal-tar derivative chemicals.

Today we are witnessing a new herbal renaissance. Chemistry-oriented modern medicine man is just beginning to realize that synthetic chemicals are poor substitutes for the *natural medicines* created by the wise God for the healing of man – the *herbs.* Our largest drug companies are spending millions of dollars searching for medicinal and rejuvenating plants on five continents. Already, effective plants and herbal remedies for the treatment of arthritis, cancer, heart troubles, asthma and mental disorders have been "rediscovered". One leading researcher at the University of Texas stated: "We've never had as much success with chemicals invented by man as we're having with plant extracts."

While most of the recent herb research is directed toward discovery of the effective natural healing substances, several teams of researchers in England, France and Russia have been investigating herbs that have an ancient reputation for preserving and restoring youth. The herbs best known for their rejuvenating properties are Ginseng, Fo-ti-Tieng, Gotu-Kola, Sarsaparilla and Damiana.

Ginseng is the most famous and the most potent rejuvenating plant. The roots of Ginseng bear a remarkable resemblance to the shape and form of man; this is why Chinese called the plant *Ginseng,* or "man-plant".

Ginseng has been used by 500 million Chinese and other people for over 5,000 years as an aphrodisiac, rejuvenator, revitalizer and cure-all for a variety of ills. If Ginseng did not produce genuine results, if its power was based on nothing but sheer superstition, don't you think man would have discarded it long before now?

The Russian Institute of Experimental Medicine made an extensive study of Ginseng and its claimed medicinal and rejuvenating properties. They discovered that Ginseng grows only in radioactive soil and that the roots of the plant itself contained many radioactive properties. They also found that the claims the Orientals were making about Ginseng were true: it strengthens the heart, revitalized the nervous system, increases hormone production, and stimulates cell growth and activity. Russians have now huge plantations of Ginseng in South Siberia. They also buy millions of dollars worth of Ginseng from Korea.

Fo-ti-Tieng, a small Oriental plant, is another well-known rejuvenator. It grows only in certain jungle districts of the Oriental tropics. Fo-ti-Tieng was popularized by the renowned Chinese herbalist, Professor Li Chung Yun, who lived to be 256 years of age. He used Fo-ti-Tieng and Ginseng daily in the form of tea. He enjoyed excellent health, outlived 23 wives, and kept his own natural teeth and hair. Those who saw him at the age of 200 testified that he did not appear much older than a man in his fifties.

British, French, and Ceylonese researchers, who made studies and clinical tests with Fo-ti-Tieng, agree that the plant contains an unknown vitamin, which they termed "vitamin X", or "the youth vitamin". This new vitamin has a rejuvenating effect on the brain cells and on the endocrine glands. The French government was so impressed by the rejuvenating properties of Fo-ti-Tieng, that it established plantations and experimental stations in Algeria.

Gotu-Kola contains rejuvenating properties similar to those of Fo-ti-Tieng and Ginseng. It grows in India, South Africa and some islands of the Indian Ocean. Gotu-Kola leaves have a marked energizing effect on the cells of the brain, and a strenghtening effect on the nerve functions. They are also used medicinally as a diuretic and kidney stimulant and a blood purifier.

But Gotu-Kola is known in the Orient primarily as a longevity plant. There are many recorded examples of unusual longevity attained by those who use Gotu-Kola regularly. It is claimed that

Gotu-Kola can add 50 years to the life span by strengthening the brain to such an extent that it will not age or break down.

Sarsaparilla is a tropical American plant that grows mostly in Honduras, Mexico, and Jamaica. The roots of the Sarsaparilla plant are used to make tea, which is used for such conditions as chronic rheumatism, skin disorders, psoriasis, general weakness and sexual impotence. Sarsaparilla is also a known blood purifer.

American and Mexican scientists discovered, independently of each other, that Sarsaparilla roots contain the male sex hormone, testosterone. Mexico and several South American countries, in fact, now manufacture testosterone tablets from Sarsaparilla. Recently, progesterone, the female sex hormone, was also discovered in Sarsaparilla roots. Even cortin, one of the adrenal hormones, was found in Sarsaparilla.

Damiana has been used by Indians in Mexico as an aphrodisiac and a general revitalizer for many centuries. So-called California Damiana is considered to be the most effective. Sarsaparilla root and Damiana are both sold by herbalists at every Mexican market.

Ginseng, Fo-ti-Tieng, Gotu-Kola, Sarsaparilla and Damiana are sold in the form of tablets, roots, or herb teas in most health food stores in the United States.

It is generally considered that the strength of the endocrine glands, and particularly of the gonads, is directly related to the general vitality and healthy functioning of the body. The sexual virility largely determines man's youthfulness, health, vitality and longevity. The decline in sex hormone production results in gradual aging and decreased life span. The effectiveness of these herbal rejuvenators is attributed to the fact that they help to keep the sex glands in peak working condition far into advanced age and, thus, help to preserve the characteristics of youth. They regenerate glandular activity and increase the production of life-giving hormones, which are the actual "fountains of youth".

ELECTRONIC OVENS

Q. *How safe are microwave ovens, also known as electronic ovens?*

A. There have been many reports of excessive radiation "leakage" and possible health hazards from some of the electronic ovens now on the market. The following warning was given by scientists in the Intelligence Branch of HEW's Division of Electronic Products:

"The potential health effects of microwave ovens are that organs of the body, such as the eyes, are unable to rapidly dissipate heat and are therefore highly vulnerable."

And a press release from HEW's Radiological Health Bureau said, in part: "Animal experiments have shown that relatively high levels of microwave radiation can cause eye cataracts and possibly other biological effects."

The National Health Federation's investigation of the alleged claims that microwave cooking retains more of the vitamins failed to find any proof to substantiate the claims. The only advantage of microwave ovens seems to be that they do cook very rapidly . But why take the risk of damaging your eyes and possibly harming your health in some other way just to save a few minutes of cooking time?

ARTHRITIS

Q. *I have been told by my doctor that there is no cure for arthritis, and I think the whole medical profession agress on that. Yet, you have written a book called THERE IS A CURE FOR ARTHRITIS. How dare you contradict the united opinion of hundreds of thousands of doctors? Or, perhaps, you know something they don't?*

A. My book has been on the market for two years and sold in six editions. You know very well that a book with such a challenging title would have been banned "sooner than quick" (and very powerful forces work continuously to accomplish just that) if it weren't truthful and 100% scientifically factual.

Contrary to what you have been told for years, there *is,* indeed, a cure for arthritis. But don't take *my* word for it. In my book you will find references to many reputable scientific studies, made by medical doctors in various countries of the world, which show that biological therapies can arrest and even cure arthritis. Several famous medical doctors collaborated with me on the book – they stand solidly behind the claim that *there is a cure for arthritis.*

An American doctor, who specialized in arthritis for years, Dr. R. P. Watterson, said, "Although not in general use, knowledge of the cause of arthritis exists, as well as measures necessary for its prevention and treatment. It is the obligation of the medical profession to recognize and use this information" (*South-Western Medicine,* April, 1961). This knowledge is presented to the public in my book. All the successful biological therapies are described in detail. Show it to your doctor and ask him why this knowledge is "not in general use", as suggested by Dr. Watterson.*

CANCER

Q. *You have mentioned in one of your books that there is a successful cancer clinic in Europe. Where is it, and how do they treat cancer there?*

A. The clinic is called Ringberg-Klinik, 8183 Rottach-Egern/ Tegernsee, West Germany. Dr. Josef Issels, M.D., is the medical director of the clinic.

The cornerstone of Dr. Issels' cancer therapy is FEVER. Artificially induced fever, plus special diets of raw foods, juices and fermented lactic-acid foods, are the most important biological treatments used at the Ringberg-Klinik.

Dr. Issels said, "Artificially induced fever has the greatest potential in the treatment of cancer."

Fever has been too long a misunderstood symptom. Fever is always instituted by the body as a positive, constructive measure in order to heal itself. It is an essential part of the body's intricate defensive and curative system. Fever:

---

*Paavo O. Airola, THERE IS A CURE FOR ARTHRITIS, Parker Publishing Co., Inc., West Nyack, New York, 1968.

- inhibits the growth of bacteria,
- speeds the metabolic processes,
- burns toxins and wastes and speeds up their elimination, and
- accelerates the healing activity.

Today's average doctor treats fever as an isolated undesirable symptom and tries to suppress it with drugs. But ancient doctors understood the real value of fever. Parmenides said 2,000 years ago, "Give me the chance to create fever and I will cure any disease."

The modern medical genius, French Nobel Prize Winner, Dr. A. Lwoff, also understood the positive character of fever. He said, "High temperature during infection helps to combat the growth of virus. Therefore fever should not be brought down with drugs."

Overheating therapies were revived by the German, Maria Schlenz, a few decades back. She wrote the now famous book, *HOW INCURABLE DISEASES ARE CURED.* Her overheating baths – the Schlenz-baths – have had most remarkable curative effect on many conditions. Famous German doctor, Professor Werner Zabel, who has his own clinic in Berchtesgaden, said, "The Schlenz-bath indeed cures incurable diseases."

Dr. Issels has achieved remarkable success with cancer patients placed on a total program of biological treatments, including overheating therapy, or artificially induced fever. Fever strengthens the body's own effort to defeat cancer, stimulates all the metabolic processes and glandular activity, and accelerates the healing activity – it literally burns up the diseased tissues and restores health.

HEALTH SECRET NO. 1

Q. *Every health writer has his own pet secret for optimum health and long life. What is yours?*

A. *Systematic undereating!* Russian statistics show that all their centenarians are moderate eaters. And Dr. C.M. McCay, of Cornell University, has demonstrated scientifically that overeating is a definite and principle cause of disease and premature aging; conversely, undereating can extend life and prevent disease. "Thin rats bury the fat rats."

We are a nation of overfed but undernourished people. Overeating results in malnutrition. Food eaten in excess of actual need acts in the system as a poison! It interferes with proper digestion and assimilation. Overeating causes fermentation, gas and putrefaction in the intestines and insufficient assimilation of nutrients. Systematic undereating will improve the digestion of foods so that all nutrients will be effectively absorbed and utilized.

No one said it better than Benjamin Franklin, when he remarked that "a full belly is the mother of all evil."

DRINKING WITH MEALS

Q. *Some authorities warn against drinking with meals – some others say that drinking with meals improves digestion. What is the real truth on this matter?*

A. I don't know of any scientific studies made on drinking with meals, but all the authorities I know and respect agree that it is better not to drink with meals. Liquids with meals will dilute the digestive juices and secretions, resulting in poor digestion of foods. Juices, water or herb teas should be drunk between meals or at least 45 to 30 minutes before meals.

RELAXATION AND PEACE OF MIND

Q. *You speak of nutrition as if it were the only important factor in health and disease. Doesn't man's mind play the decisive role?*

A. I am a nutritionist and, consequently, my lectures and books deal with the nutritional aspects of health. This is what the listeners and the readers expect to learn from a nutritionist. This does not mean, however, that I minimize the importance of man's mind as a decisive factor in health and disease. Indeed, "As a man thinketh in his heart, so he is."

I believe that relaxation and peace of mind are very important health-promoting factors, perhaps the most important. These are what modern man needs most of all in order to live a long and happy life in good health.

It has been scientifically established that emotional stresses and disturbances can cause practically every disease in the medical dictionary, including arthritis, ulcers, constipation, asthma, strokes, diabetes, high or low blood pressure, angina, glandular disturbances, etc. Extensive research into medical literature made by J. I. Rodale indicates that "happy people rarely get cancer". Unhappiness, deprivation of love, loneliness, constant fear, anxiety, depression, worries – all these emotional stresses and tensions can interfere with your normal body functions and may lead to serious illness.

There are many factors that contribute to optimum health. Nutrition is *one* very important factor. But relaxation, peace of mind, positive outlook on life, contented spirit, absence of envy and jealousy, cheerful disposition, love of mankind and faith in God – these are all powerful, health-promoting factors without which optimum health can not be achieved.

Perhaps I should add here that all the endeavors for attaining better physical health would be wasted unless the healthy body is used as a worthy temple for the spirit to dwell in and develop. The purpose of life is not just the building of a magnificent body, or living a long life, but perfecting and refining our divine spirit and becoming more God-like. The real purpose of having good health is to prepare a way for our spiritual growth and perfection.

Chapter 16

Recipes & Directions

FOR SPECIAL FOODS RECOMMENDED IN THIS BOOK

Below are recipes and directions for preparing special dishes, salads, breads and other health and longevity foods named and recommended in this book. Most of the ingredients mentioned in the recipes are available at better health food stores.

WAERLAND FIVE-GRAIN KRUSKA

(for 4 persons)

1 tbsp. whole wheat
1 tbsp. whole rye
1 tbsp. whole barley
1 tbsp. whole millet
1 tbsp. whole oats
2 tbsp. wheat bran
2 tbsp. unsulphured raisins

Take five grains and grind them coarsely on your own grinder. Place in a pot with one to one and a half cups of water and add bran and raisins. Boil for five to ten minutes, then wrap the pot in a blanket or newspapers and let it stand for a few hours. Experiment with the amount of water used – kruska must not be mushy, but should have the consistency of a very thick porridge.

Serve hot with sweet milk and homemade applesauce or stewed fruits.

Kruska is an extremely nutritious dish and should be taken as a meal in itself.

UNCOOKED QUICK KRUSKA

Use the same ingredients as above. Pour boiling water over freshly ground grains and other ingredients and let stand and steep for about half an hour. This Quick Kruska is delicious and more easily digestible because of the preserved enzymes. Serve warm and eat the same way as the cooked Five-grain Kruska.

HOMEMADE APPLESAUCE

Use only unsprayed apples. Sprayed apples should be carefully brushed and washed or peeled. Cut up whole apples – peel, core and all – and stew in a small quantity of water until soft. Use a stainless steel utensil and only enough water to cover the bottom. Sweeten with honey, if necessary. If the apples are sweet, no sweetening is needed. When apples are soft, pass them through a sieve or blend in a blender. Keep in refrigerator.

FRUIT SALAD À LA AIROLA

1 bowl fresh fruits, organically grown if possible
1 handful raw nuts and/or sunflower seeds
3-4 soaked prunes or handful of raisins, unsulphured
3 tbsp. cottage cheese, preferably homemade, unsalted
1 tbsp. raw wheat germ, only if you can buy it fresh
3 tbsp. yogurt
1 tbsp. wheat germ oil
2 tsp. natural, unpasteurized honey
1 tsp. fresh lemon juice

Wash all fruits carefully and dry. Use any available fruits and berries, but try to get at least three or four different kinds. Peaches, grapes, pears, papaya, bananas, strawberries, and fresh pineapple are particularly good for producing a delightful bouquet of rich, penetrating flavors. A variety of colors will make the salad festive and attractive to the eye.

Chop or slice bigger fruits, but leave grapes and berries whole. Place them in a large bowl and add prunes and nuts (nuts and sunflower seeds could be crushed). Make a dressing with one teaspoon honey (or more if most of the fruits used are sour), one teaspoon of lemon juice, and two tablespoons of water. Pour over the fruit, add wheat germ, and toss well. Mix cottage cheese, yogurt, wheat germ oil, and one teaspoon of honey in a separate cup until it is fairly smooth in texture and pour it on top of the salad. Sprinkle with nuts and sunflower seeds. Serve at once.

This is not only a most delicious dish but it is the most nutritious and perfectly balanced meal I know. It is a storehouse of high-grade proteins and all the essential vitamins, minerals, fatty acids and enzymes you need for optimum health. This salad should be a daily *must* for the beauty-conscious and health-conscious alike.

KASHA
(buckwheat cereal)

1 cup whole buckwheat grains

2 cups water

Bring water to a boil. Stir the buckwheat into the boiling water and let boil for two to three minutes. Turn heat to low and simmer for 15 to 20 minutes, stirring occasionally. If seasoning is desired use a very little sea salt. When all the water is absorbed, take from the stove and let stand for another 15 minutes. Kasha must never be mushy. Serve hot with sunflower seed oil or butter.

This is a favorite cereal in Russia and many other Eastern European countries. It has an unusual mellow flavor and it is extremely nutritious.

MILLET CEREAL

1 cup hulled millet

3 cups water

½ tsp. honey

½ cup powdered skim milk

Rinse millet in warm water and drain. Place in a pan of water mixed with powdered skim milk and heat mixture to boiling point. Then simmer for ten minutes, stirring occasionally to prevent sticking and burning. Remove from heat and let stand for a half hour or more. Serve with milk, honey, oil, or butter – or homemade applesauce! And treat yourself to the *most nutritious cereal in the world!*

MOLINO CEREAL

1 tbsp. coarse whole wheat flour
2 tbsp. wheat bran
2 tbsp. whole flaxseed
2-3 chopped figs or soaked prunes, or
1 tbsp. unsulphured raisins

Place all the ingredients in a pan with one cup of water and boil for five minutes, stirring occasionally to prevent burning. Serve immediately with sweet milk, a little honey, or homemade applesauce.

This cereal is served in European clinics to patients with weak digestion and a tendency toward constipation.

POTATO CEREAL

2 large raw potatoes
2 tbsp. whole wheat flour
1 tbsp. wheat bran
1 tbsp. wheat germ
4 cups water

Heat water to boiling point. Mix flour and bran in pan and simmer for two to three minutes. Place a fine shredder over pan and quickly shred potatoes directly into pan. Stir vigorously and lift from the stove. Let stand for a few minutes and serve hot with milk, butter, or cream; sprinkle wheat germ on top.

This is an alkaline and exceptionally nutritious cereal. It is used often in Swedish biological clinics, especially in diets for patients with rheumatic diseases.

RUSSIAN BORSCH

beets, cabbage, potatoes, tomato
onions, sour cream, young beet leaves,
fresh dill, chives, bay leaf

Boil cabbage, potatoes, onions, beets and bay leaf until soft. Add tomato and simmer for 2 minutes. Serve with sour cream and chopped dill, beet tops and chives on top. A dash of sea salt may be used for seasoning.

RUSSIAN SUMMER BORSCH

After you make your homemade cottage cheese (see recipe in this chapter) save the liquid whey and store in refrigerator. For a delicious and refreshing lunch on a hot summer day, fill the plate with whey and chop in cold cooked potatoes and beets, fresh tomatoes, dill, chives and a little sour pickle or sauerkraut. Serve with a dab of sour cream on top.

SPROUTED WHEAT

There are many different methods of sprouting seeds. Waerland recommends the following method: soak the wheat grains in water at room temperature for three nights and spread them thinly on a dish or paper towel for three days. To prevent the grains from molding they must be rinsed under running water three times a day. When the sprouts are the length of the seed they are ready for eating.

Another good method is to soak wheat overnight in cold water, then roll the scattered seeds inside a wet clean towel. Sprinkle water over the towel several times a day.

Sprouted beans and seeds are excellent health foods, and everyone can benefit by using them regularly.

HALVAH

1 cup sesame seeds

2 tsp. honey, preferably coagulated solid honey

Grind sesame seeds on a small electric seed grinder. Pour sesame meal into a larger cup and knead honey into the meal with a large spoon until honey is well mixed and the halvah acquires the consistency of a hard dough. Serve as it is, or make small balls and roll them in whole sesame seeds, shredded coconut, or sunflower seeds.

HOMEMADE SOURED MILK

Use only unpasteurized, raw milk. Place a bottle of milk in a pan filled with warm water and warm it to about body temperature. Fill a cup or a deep plate, stir in tablespoon of yogurt, cover with paper towel (for dust) and keep in warm place – for example, near the stove, heating radiator, or wherever there is a constant warm temperature. The milk will coagulate in approximately 24 hours.

Use one or two spoonfuls of soured milk as a culture for your next batch (use yogurt or commercial buttermilk only as a starting culture for the first batch.)

HOMEMADE COTTAGE CHEESE

Take homemade soured milk and warm it to about 140° F – but not higher than 160° F (70° C) – by placing the container in warm water. When the milk has curdled, place a clean linen canvas over a deep strainer and pour curdled milk over it. Wait until all liquid whey has seeped through the strainer. What remains in the strainer is fresh, wholesome, and delicious homemade cottage cheese. If the cheese is too hard, add a little sweet or sour cream, and stir. The higher the temperature the harder the cheese, and vice versa.

By the way, don't throw the whey away – it is an exceptionally nutritious, beautifying and rejuvenating drink.

HOMEMADE YOGURT

Take a bottle of skim milk and heat it almost to boiling, then cool to room temperature. Add two to three tablespoons of yogurt, which can be bought in a grocery store or health shop. Stir well. Pour into a wide-mouthed thermos bottle. Cover and let it stand overnight. In five to eight hours it will be solid and ready to serve. If you do not have a thermos jar, use an ordinary glass jar, and place it in a pan of warm water over an electric burner switched on "warm" for four to five hours, then switch off until milk is solid.

Use two to three spoonfuls of your fresh, homemade yogurt as a culture for the next batch.

PAPAYA SPLIT

½ papaya, chilled
1 cup yogurt
2 tsp. liquid honey
1 tbsp. sunflower or pumpkin seeds

Cut whole papaya in half. Remove seeds. Mix honey and yogurt well and then fill the hollow papaya with the mixture. Sprinkle seeds on top.

This is my own recipe, and everyone who tries it compliments me on it. It is a satisfying, extremely nourishing, mild, cleansing, and very easily digestible dish – and most delicious, too.

SWEDISH ROSE HIP SOUP

Take two tablespoons of rose hip powder for each cup of water or for each serving. Boil in pan for five minutes. Sweeten with honey and thicken with a half-tablespoon of corn starch or potato flour per serving. Soybean flour can also be used to make the soup even more nutritious. After adding the thickening, boil again for three minutes. Serve warm or chilled. Can be served with sweet milk or cream, and sprinkled with wheat germ, crushed raw nuts, or sunflower seeds. An excellent, nutritious dessert!

ROSE HIP TEA

Take one tablespoon of dried rose hips or rose hip powder for each cup of water. Bring to a boil, but do not actually boil, then steep for five minutes (for powder) or 15 minutes (for whole or halves). Strain, sweeten with honey, and enjoy a vitamin C-loaded, nutritious and beautifying pink-colored tea. Imported Scandinavian rose hips and rose hip powder can be bought in health food stores, even in the United States.

Note: do not use aluminum utensils when cooking rose hips!

SOUR RYE BREAD
(Black Bread Russian Style)

8 cups freshly ground whole rye flour
3 cups warm water
½ cup sourdough culture

Mix seven cups of flour with water and sourdough culture. Cover and let stand in a warm place overnight between 12 and 18 hours. Add remaining flour and mix well. Place in greased pans. Let it rise for approximately a half-hour. Bake at 350° F, one hour or more, if needed. Always save a half-cup of dough as a culture for the next baking. Keep the culture in a tight jar in your refrigerator. For the initial baking it will be necessary to obtain a sourdough culture from a commercial baker.

This recipe makes 2 two-pound loaves.

HOMEMADE SAUERKRAUT

Use a small wooden barrel, or a large earthenware pot. Possibly a large stainless steel pail or a glass jar could be used, but under no circumstances use an aluminum utensil.

Cut white cabbage heads into narrow strips with a large knife or grater, and place in a barrel. When the layer of cabbage is about four to six inches deep, sprinkle a few juniper berries, cummin seeds and/or black currant leaves on top – use your favorite or whatever you have available. A few strips of carrots, beets, green peppers, and onions can also be used. Add a little sea salt - not more than two ounces for each 25 pounds of cabbage. (Sauerkraut can also be made without salt.) Then add another layer of grated cabbage and spices until the container is filled. Each layer should be pressed and stamped very hard with your fists or a piece of wood so that there will be no air left and the cabbage will be saturated with its own juice.

When the container is full, cover cabbage with a clean linen canvas, place a wooden or slate board over it, and on the top place a clean heavy stone. Let stand for three to four weeks in a warm place, not below 70° F. Now and then remove the foam and the possible mildew from the top, from the stone and from the barrel edges. The linen canvas, board and stone should be occasionally removed, washed well with warm water and then cold water, and replaced. After three to four weeks the sauerkraut is ready for eating. It can be left in the barrel, which now should be stored in a cool place, or put in glass jars and kept in the refrigerator.

Sauerkraut is best eaten *raw* – both from the point of taste and for its health-giving value. Drink sauerkraut juice, too. It is an extremely beneficial and wonderfully nutritious drink.

HOMEMADE PICKLED VEGETABLES (or lactic acid vegetables)

Use the same method as described above for homemade sauerkraut to make health-giving lactic acid vegetables. Beets, carrots, green and red peppers, beet tops, swiss chard, and celery are particularly adapted for pickling.

HOMEMADE SOUR PICKLES

Use only small, fresh, hard cucumbers. Place them in cold water overnight, then dry them well.

Place cucumbers in a wooden barrel, or a large earthenware, or glass jar. Place a few leaves of black currants, cherries, mustard seeds and dill branches in with the cucumbers.

Boil up a sufficient amount of salt water, using about four ounces of sea salt for five quarts of water. Let water cool down, then pour it over cucumbers. Cover with linen canvas, place a wooden board over it, and on the top a clean heavy stone. There should be enough salt water to cover the board. Keep container in a warm place for about one week, then move to a cooler place. Pickles are ready for eating in about three to four weeks. Every second week or so remove the stone and the covers and wash them well, first in warm then in cold water; then replace them. Keep the top of the water clean from foam and mildew. When pickles are ready for eating they can be placed in glass jars and kept in the refrigerator.

Index

F

G

H

I

J

K

L

ABOUT THE AUTHOR

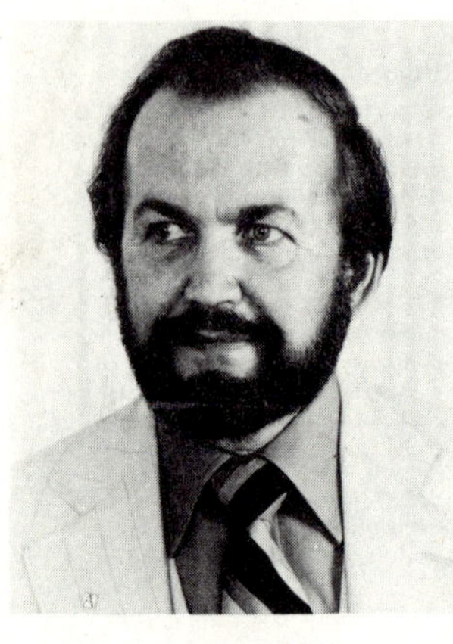

Paavo Airola, Ph.D., N.D., is an internationally recognized nutritionist, naturopathic physician, lecturer, and an award-winning author. He studied nutrition, biochemistry, and biological medicine in Europe and spent many years of research and study in European biological clinics and research centers. He is considered to be the leading authority on biological medicine and wholistic approach to healing in the United States. He lectures extensively, and worldwide, both to professionals and laymen, holding yearly educational seminars for physicians. He has recently lectured at the Stanford University Medical School.

Dr. Airola is the author of eleven widely-read books, notably his two international best-sellers, ***Are You Confused?*** and ***How To Get Well.*** The American Academy of Public Affairs issued Dr. Airola the Award of Merit for his book, ***There Is A Cure For Arthritis. Are You Confused?*** is heralded by many nutritionists, doctors, and critics as "the most important health book ever published," "a must reading for every sincere health seeker."

His comprehensive handbook on natural healing, ***How To Get Well,*** is the most authoritative and practical manual on biological medicine in print. It outlines complete nutritional, herbal, and other alternative biological therapies for all of our most common ailments and is used as a textbook in several universities and medical schools. It is regarded as a reliable reference manual by doctors, researchers, nutritionists, and students of health, nutrition, and biological medicine.

Dr. Airola's newest book, ***Hypoglycemia: A Better Approach,*** has revolutionized the concept of and the therapeutic approach to this insidious, complex, and devastating affliction which has assumed epidemic proportions.

Dr. Airola is President of the International Academy of Biological Medicine; a member of the International Naturopathic Association; and a member of the International Society for Research on Civilization Diseases and Environment, the prestigious forum for world-wide research, founded by Dr. Albert Schweitzer. He is listed in ***The Directory of International Biography, The Blue Book, The Men of Achievement, Who's Who In American Art,*** and ***Who's Who in the West.***